PENGUIN BOOKS

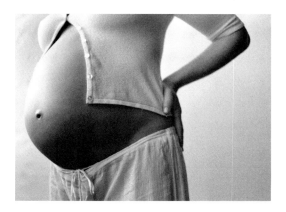

The Pregnant Body

I had great pleasure in reviewing this simple but effective guide to the aches and pains of pregnancy. Dorothy Gliksman has explained very clearly and with excellent illustrations many of the common problems found in pregnancy. It is a very simple but practical guide for women to help them overcome the minor aches and pains. Women will find this a very useful and commonsense approach with a sound medical base to alleviate many of their complaints. It certainly fills a gap that is not covered by any other publication.

Dr Wendy L. Cox
MB, BS, FRACOG, DDU
Obstetrician and Gynaecologist

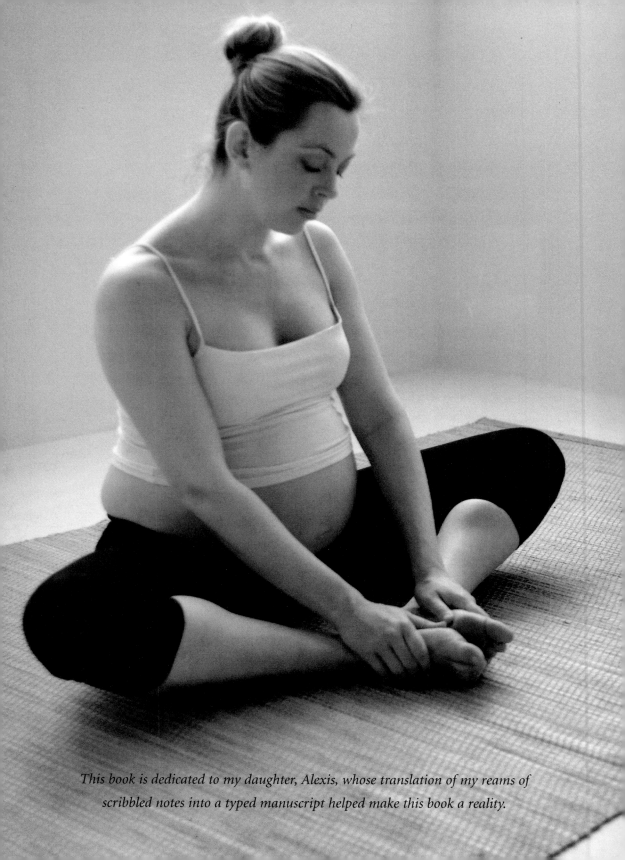

This book is dedicated to my daughter, Alexis, whose translation of my reams of scribbled notes into a typed manuscript helped make this book a reality.

The Pregnant Body

simple exercises to ease the common discomforts of pregnancy

dorothy gliksman

PENGUIN BOOKS

Penguin Books

Published by the Penguin Group
Penguin Books Australia Ltd
250 Camberwell Road, Camberwell, Victoria 3124, Australia
Penguin Books Ltd
80 Strand, London WC2R 0RL, England
Penguin Putnam Inc.
375 Hudson Street, New York, New York 10014, USA
Penguin Books Canada Limited
10 Alcorn Avenue, Toronto, Ontario, Canada M4V 3B2
Penguin Books (NZ) Ltd
Cnr Rosedale and Airborne Roads, Albany, Auckland, New Zealand
Penguin Books (South Africa) (Pty) Ltd
24 Sturdee Avenue, Rosebank, Johannesburg 2196, South Africa
Penguin Books India (P) Ltd
11, Community Centre, Panchsheel Park, New Delhi 110 017, India

First published by Penguin Books Australia Ltd 2002

10 9 8 7 6 5 4 3 2 1

Cover design by Louise Leffler and Irma Schick, Penguin Design Studio
Text design by Louise Leffler, Penguin Design Studio
Typeset in 10.5 pt Univers Light by Post Pre-press Group, Brisbane, Queensland
Text separations by Splitting Image Colour Studio Pty Ltd, Clayton, Victoria
Printed and bound in Singapore by Imago Productions

National Library of Australia
Cataloguing-in-Publication data:

Gliksman, Dorothy.
The pregnant body

Includes index.
ISBN 0 14 026559 7.

1. Pregnancy – Popular works. 2. Pregnant women. I. Title.

618.24

www.penguin.com.au

contents

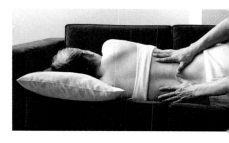

8   massage for pregnant bodies

9   relaxation for delivery

10   life after childbirth

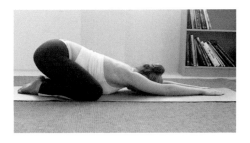

foreword

Pregnancy is generally considered a time of great joy, anticipation and excitement, and there is considerable attention given to the mother-to-be by her family and friends. However, pregnant women often also have to deal with conflicting advice from well-meaning relatives and friends about how best to care for themselves, as well as an underlying fear of possible adverse outcomes from the pregnancy, and a series of persistent and irritating minor complaints that can detract from the joy of pregnancy.

This book is not intended as an obstetric text, nor a major work on childbirth education. It can more readily be described as a book containing easy-to-follow advice on how to get the best out of pregnancy, how to avoid some of the complications and how to deal with a wide variety of problems that occur during pregnancy.

Dorothy Gliksman has had a long and close association with pregnant women as a childbirth educator and physiotherapist with special interest in women's health. This gives her the authority, based on her personal experience and knowledge of the evidence for what works to improve outcomes, to produce this concise book. *The Pregnant Body* is packed with sound advice and easy exercises that will help to make your pregnancy a more satisfying experience.

Dr Andrew Child
Head, Department of Obstetrics
King George V Memorial Hospital for Mothers and Babies
Sydney

preface

Walk into any bookshop and you will find countless books on pregnancy and childbirth, offering advice on what to do and what not to do, before, during and after childbirth. It's not my intention to add to them. This book is about you, the mother-to-be, your body and how to recognise, prevent, or cope effectively with the aches and pains associated with pregnancy.

As you experience the normal, natural stages of pregnancy, you will usually develop aches, pains and discomfort at some point. These 'normal' aches and pains are the focus of this book, along with appropriate hints and advice to ease the resultant discomfort.

If you experience any unusual, acute pain, or any bleeding, you should see your doctor immediately. If your doctor advises you that your pain is just 'one of those things' associated with pregnancy, the advice and simple exercises in this book will be indispensable in ensuring that your pregnancy will be as painless and enjoyable as possible.

This book is a culmination of over 15 years' experience in working with pregnant women as a women's health physiotherapist, treating, advising and running pregnancy fitness classes. For years, women have come to me with complaints of everything from backache to insomnia. Often they are quite distressed and believe that they have to put up with a problem since it is 'just part of life as a pregnant woman'. But simply being able to recognise the most common aches and pains and learning some basic techniques for relieving them is often the key to enjoying a far more comfortable pregnancy. Sometimes it's as easy as learning how to stretch properly, or how to change your sitting or standing posture that makes all the difference. Seeing the dramatic changes a straightforward piece of advice can provide for a pregnant woman's day-to-day life is the reason I take such joy in writing this book.

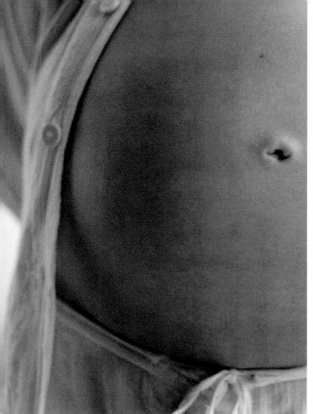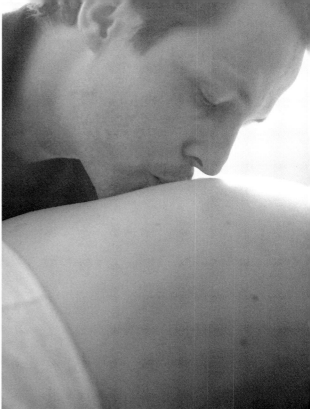

This is not a complex medical tome that will inundate you with information you won't need to know; it is an easy-to-read, informative guide to recognising and managing the common discomforts of pregnancy and beyond. Instead of wading through all sorts of advice in magazines and medical booklets, follow these suggestions and take your first step towards fully enjoying your pregnancy.

You can read this book either by starting at the beginning and reading it through, or go straight to the section that applies to you at this particular time, whether it's to find exercises to help ease upper back pain, or to learn how to stand and sit properly.

The advice contained in this book is also preventative, so reading it from start to finish will arm you with information and techniques so that you can avoid problems before they begin.

acknowledgements

My thanks go to all those people who helped me turn my experiences into this book. To Julie Gibbs, Executive Publisher at Penguin Books, who saw the need for such a book in the pregnancy field; my editors, Jacquie Brown and Jane Morrow, and designer, Louise Leffler, for guiding me so well; Rob Fisher, the talented photographer; Laura Dominique, the hair and make-up artist; as well as my two lovely models, Natalie Ewen and Donna Goram.

Thank you also to my hundreds of patients, without whose varied experiences this book would not have been possible. And thank you to Dr Andrew Child, Head of the Department of Obstetrics at King George V Memorial Hospital for Mothers and Babies, and Dr Wendy Cox, MB, BS, FRACOG, DDU, for their encouragement and assistance.

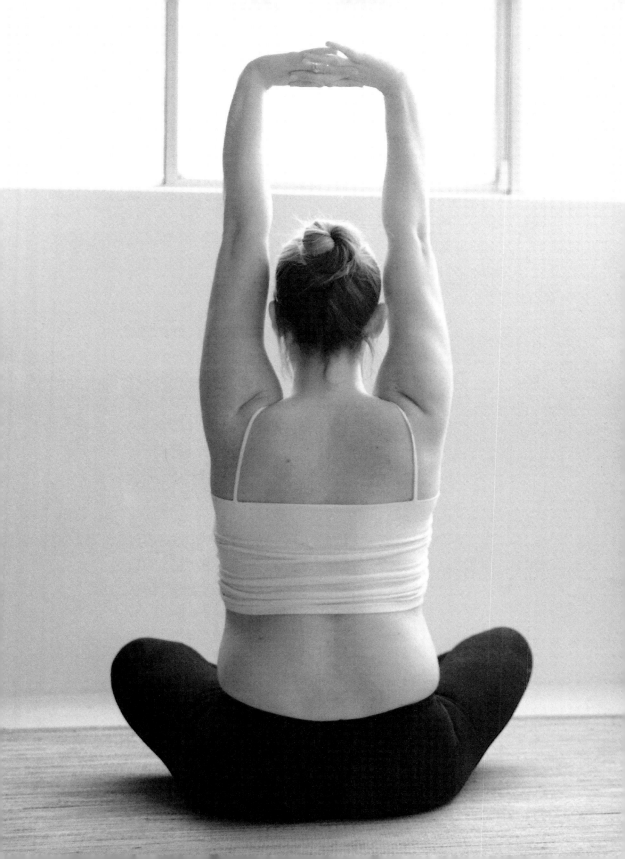

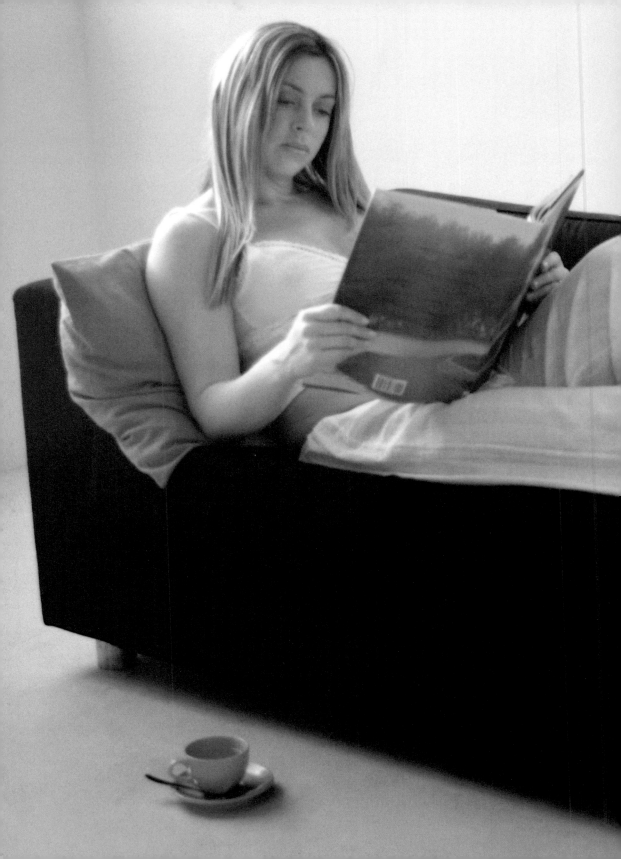

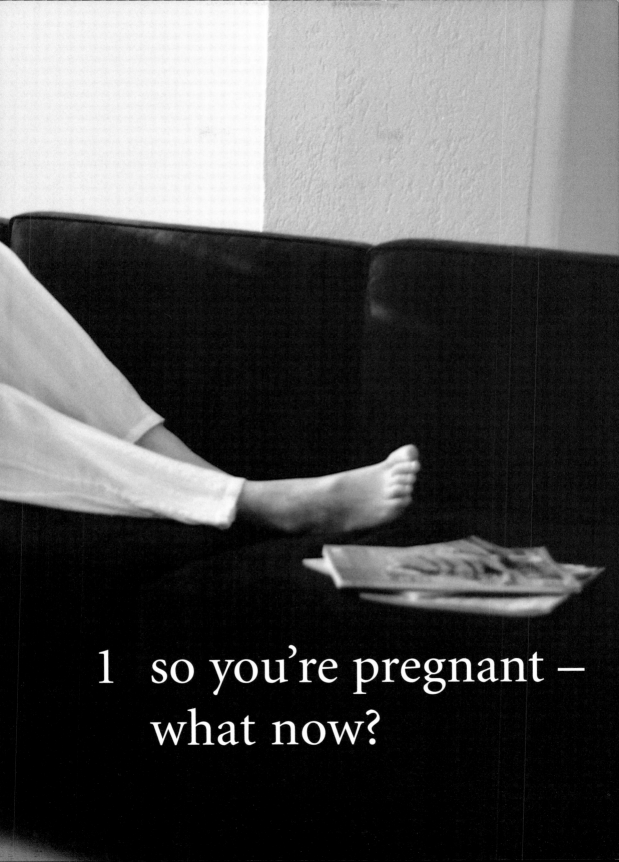

1 so you're pregnant –
what now?

tummy changes

As your pregnancy progresses, all you probably see when you look at yourself is your belly growing bigger. But inside your body, all sorts of amazing things are happening to accommodate your growing baby. The diagrams on pages 4 and 5 show the internal organs before and during pregnancy. Look at the difference! Have you ever wondered what will happen to your stomach and its muscles, your bladder, intestines, lungs and spine now that you're pregnant? Where do they go to make room for the growing uterus – and your growing baby? Learning about the wonders of the body's reproductive system is one of the joys of pregnancy, both for you and your partner.

Your uterus is normally the size of a clenched fist and the shape of a pear. Over the nine months of pregnancy, it grows into a large, hard structure and takes up most of the space in your expanding belly.

You begin to experience upward pressure on your stomach and lungs. There is downward pressure on your bladder and pelvis; outward against your abdominal muscles; and pulling on the ligaments that attach your uterus to your body – not to mention the strain on your back and groin. Is it any wonder that you may experience aches, pains and discomfort during this process!

This is your baby, growing, week by week. This miraculous event is happening inside your body. Imagining your baby taking shape and your body working around it will help you become aware of these changes and this awareness will help you to recognise and handle the accompanying discomfort effectively.

As your uterus pushes upwards as your baby grows, you will most likely experience indigestion and heartburn and you may feel breathless when walking or exercising. This is normal.

With the downward pressure of your uterus you will experience pressure in the pelvic area and on your bladder – you will be running off to the loo quite often during the day and night. Again, this is normal. And as your uterus pushes outwards, your abdominal muscles lengthen and they may separate down the centre (see page 36 for information on abdominal separation).

As your uterus keeps growing, the ligaments attaching it to your body stretch and at times you may feel a sharp, stitch-like sensation in your groin, especially if you move quickly from one position to another, or if you have been walking too quickly or for a long time. Your rapidly enlarging uterus also causes changes in your posture and your centre of gravity and at times you may feel off balance. Throughout your pregnancy, try to remember to slow down: this is one way of assisting your body as it undergoes these changes.

As incredible as all these changes can seem at the time, rest assured, they are normal. And each woman will experience the changes to her body very differently.

Rest assured, too, that as you grow, your size and shape is the right one for you. It's important not to compare yourself with someone else who may be at the same stage of pregnancy, as there are many factors that determine your size – the size of your baby is just one of them. Whatever size and shape you are, provided you are eating sensibly and exercising, is the appropriate size for you.

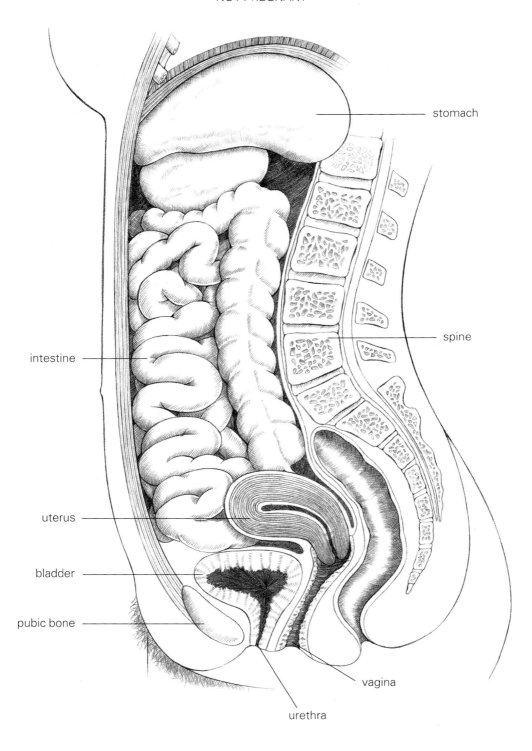

stomach

spine

intestine

uterus

bladder

pubic bone

vagina

urethra

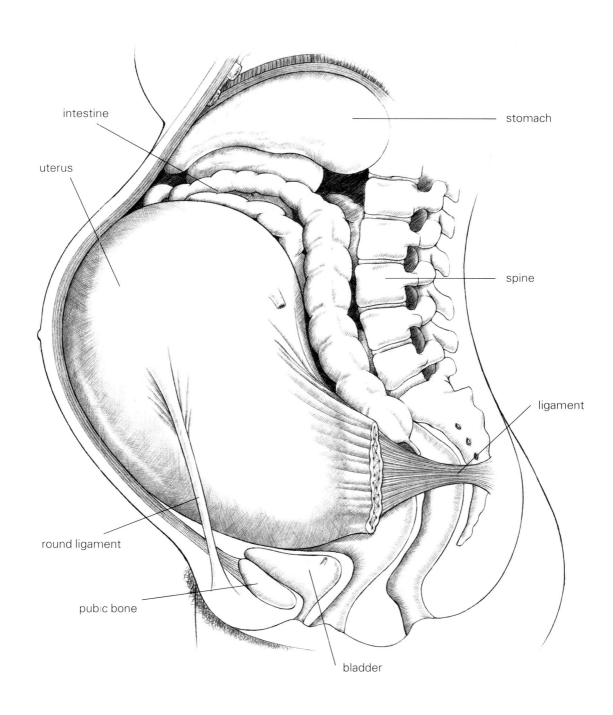

intestine

stomach

uterus

spine

ligament

round ligament

pubic bone

bladder

hormonal changes

Hormones are responsible for most of the changes your body goes through during pregnancy, such as the softening of ligaments and connective tissues and joint laxity. Hormones give the signals that prepare your body to stimulate these changes.

The downside to all these hormonal changes is that they can be the cause of some discomfort. It's common to experience forgetfulness, swollen feet and legs, heartburn or reflux and carpal tunnel syndrome, to name a few. The hormone relaxin, which begins to appear in your body after conception, along with other hormonal changes, can contribute to pelvic pain, lower and upper back pain, groin pain and the sometimes debilitating pubic symphysitis. Provided the aches and pains you experience have been checked by your obstetric carer and are not due to any serious underlying factors, there are steps you can take to ease these discomforts. See Chapter 7 for information on these conditions and advice on how to alleviate them.

Opposite and over are some of the most common complaints experienced during pregnancy. Do you relate to any of them? If you do, you are not alone. These are normal, hormone-related conditions experienced by pregnant women, and reading this book is your first step towards helping ease your discomfort.

Never feel you are wasting your doctor's, midwife's or physiotherapist's time, or that your concerns or questions may be silly or trivial. Always express your concerns; after all, this is a very special time in your life and your health and that of your baby are the most important considerations.

Forgetfulness

I thought I was going mad; I would begin to do or get something when halfway through I'd completely forget what I was meant to do. Keys – forget that! I was forever forgetting where I'd put them. Not only that, I also found I was very emotional for no reason – the slightest thing would make me cry and I would get upset with my partner over very little.
– Judy, 32 weeks, first baby

Swollen feet and legs

Towards the end of the day, my feet and legs were not only quite enlarged, but aching as well. I had to increase my shoe size at around 30 weeks.
– Gayle, 38 weeks, second baby

Heartburn/reflux

Nights were the worst. I couldn't lie down without getting a burning sensation in my upper chest. I was bringing up wind quite a bit, too. My doctor suggested buying one of those indigestion products suitable for pregnancy from the chemist and she gave me other advice on eating ginger and drinking peppermint tea, which also helped.
– Natalie, 26 weeks, first baby

Carpal tunnel syndrome

My hands and arms are swollen and painful; my right hand is worse than my left. I also feel tingling and numbness in my hands and fingers. I can't sleep at night and I'm afraid to hold a cup – I'm worried I might drop it.
– Jane, 35 weeks, first baby

Pelvic pain

I thought the aches in my hips and lower back were due to straining myself after shopping one day. My physiotherapist explained it was due to the loosening of certain ligaments and the way I was sitting.

– Jane, 32 weeks, first baby

Lower back pain

When I started to have back pain at 21 weeks I thought it was going to last or get worse, but after understanding the reasons for the pain, then changing the way I sat or did the housework, my pain gradually decreased and disappeared altogether.

– Sally, 25 weeks, first baby

Upper back pain

After only a couple of hours in front of the computer, I started to get a sharp pain between my shoulder blades. I thought I would have to stop work and I had planned to continue for another month at least. After being shown some very simple exercises, my pain became a lot better.

– Faye, 28 weeks, second baby

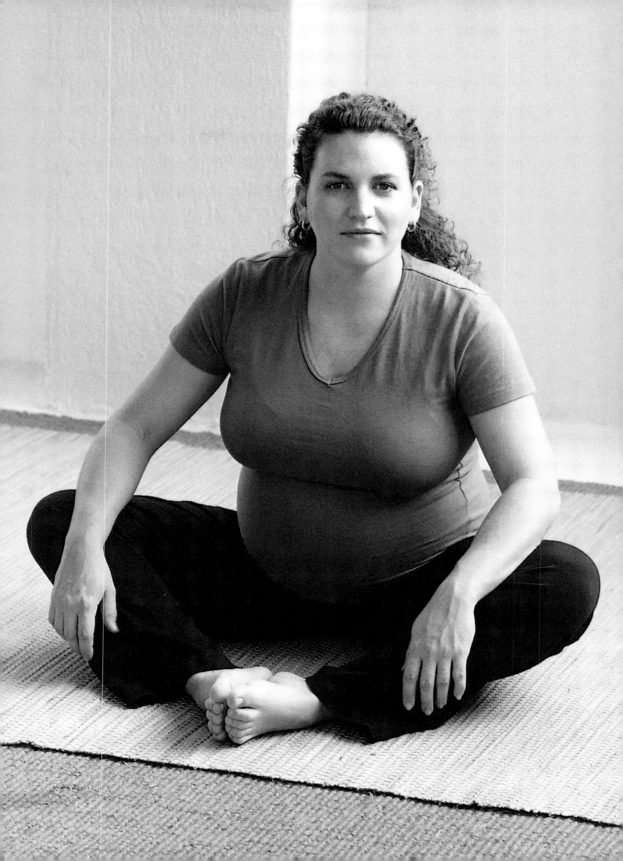

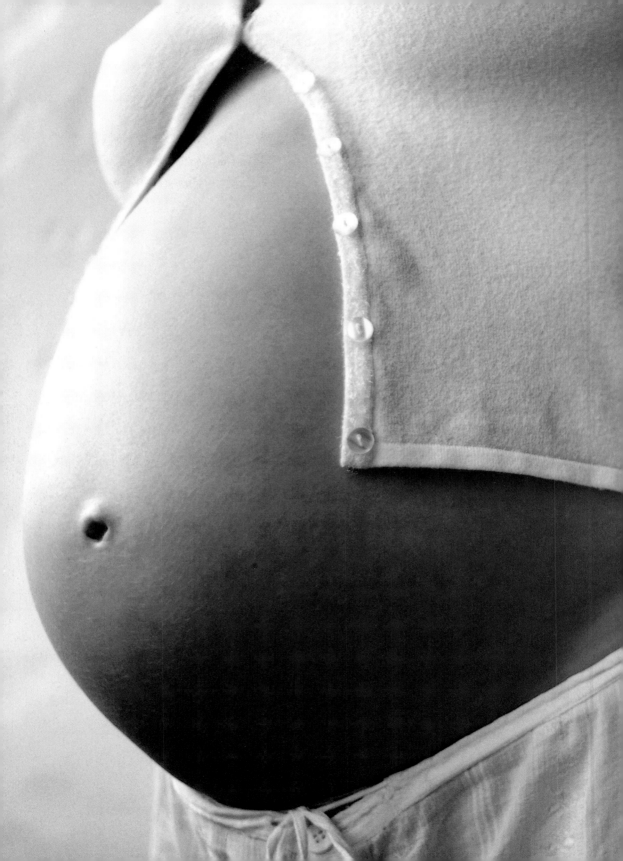

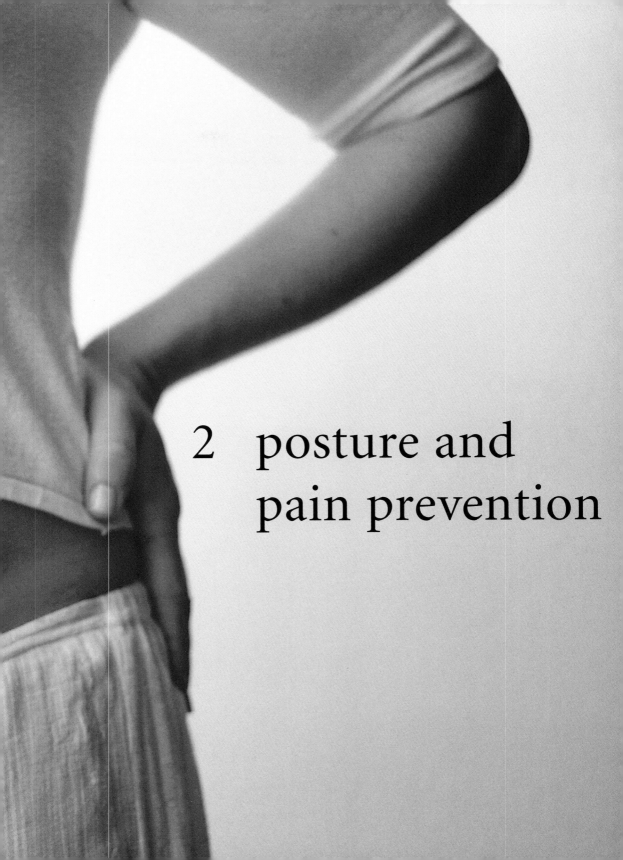

2   posture and
pain prevention

good posture

During pregnancy your ligaments, muscles and joints soften, so it is very important to be aware of your posture. It is easy to round your shoulders and stick your tummy out, but it is just as easy not to.

As it grows, the uterus pulls on the spine, which can tend to create a 'sway-back' shape and cause you to waddle as you walk. Penguins walk this way, you don't have to!

Be aware of this tendency to pull forward with your spine and modify your posture. There are three important points for good posture:

- tummy in
- shoulders back
- bottom tucked under

Remember these three points, whatever you are doing – whether you are sitting, standing or walking. Maintaining good posture will go a long way in preventing and eliminating backache. (And yes, you can pull your tummy muscles in when you are pregnant!)

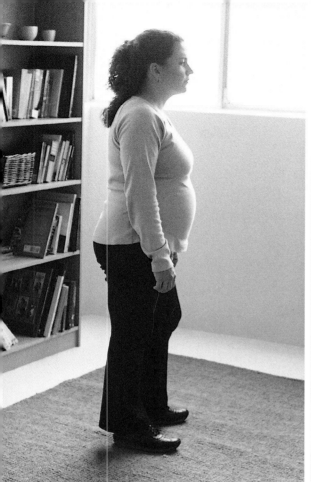

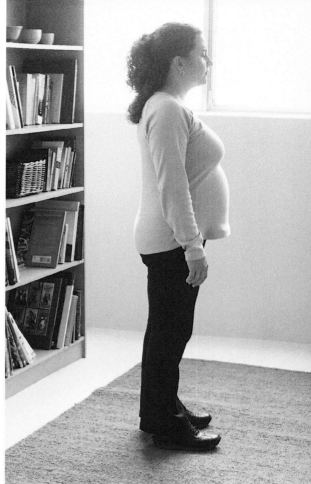

Incorrect standing posture – slumped   *Correct postural alignment*

The penguin waddle – how often have you seen pregnant women with that walk? Imagine carrying a watermelon strapped to your tummy – you can either be weighed down by it or you can carry it strongly and properly.

sitting

The worst sitting position when you are pregnant is slumped into a soft sofa. This puts tremendous strain on your lower back, as there is no support, and doesn't do your joints any good.

Always make sure you sit upright, with your lower back well supported. Sit in an upright chair with your back straight, or place a pillow behind your lower back if you're sitting in a soft chair. For added comfort, rest your feet on a stool.

An excellent way of sitting, which is both comfortable and sensible, is to sit on the floor or on your bed in the positions described in the next few pages, keeping your back straight. Having your knees bent will help support your back in these positions when you are relaxing, for example, reading a book, watching television or listening to music. Not only will these positions help you prepare your body for labour, they are beneficial for your back.

Having strong muscles, and being aware of your posture as your body changes and the weight you are carrying increases, can make a huge difference to how you look, move and feel.

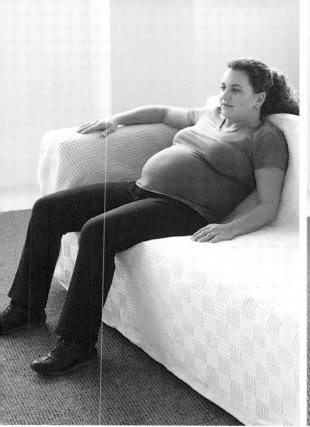

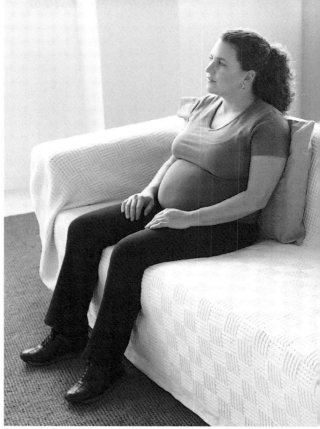

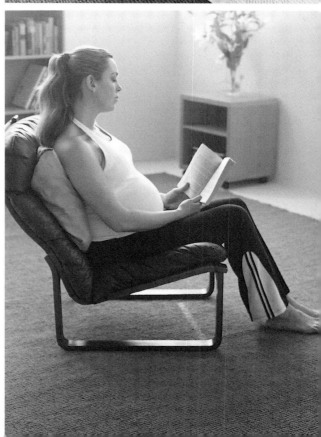

Above left: A slumped sitting position will lead to backache

Above right: A good, supported sitting position will help prevent backache

Right: A supported, comfortable, relaxed sitting position

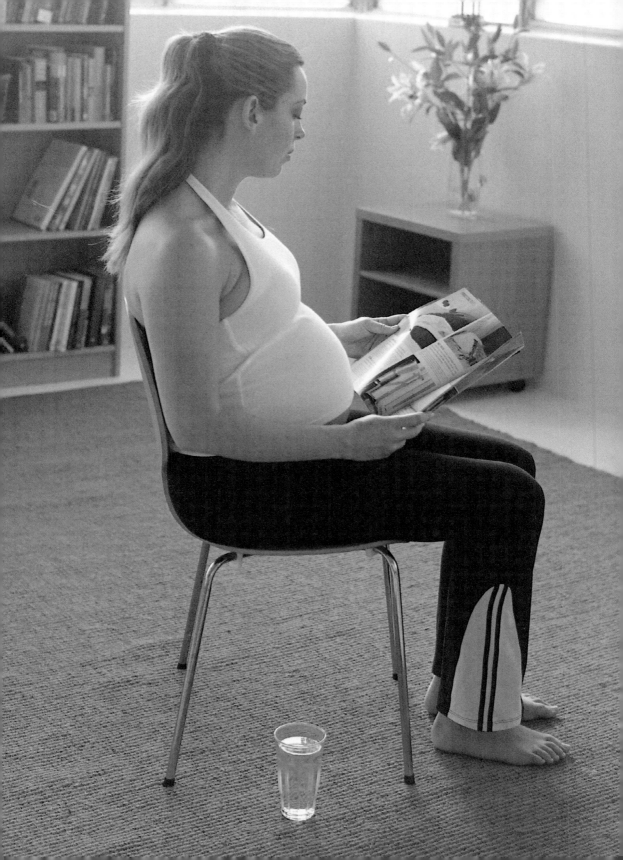

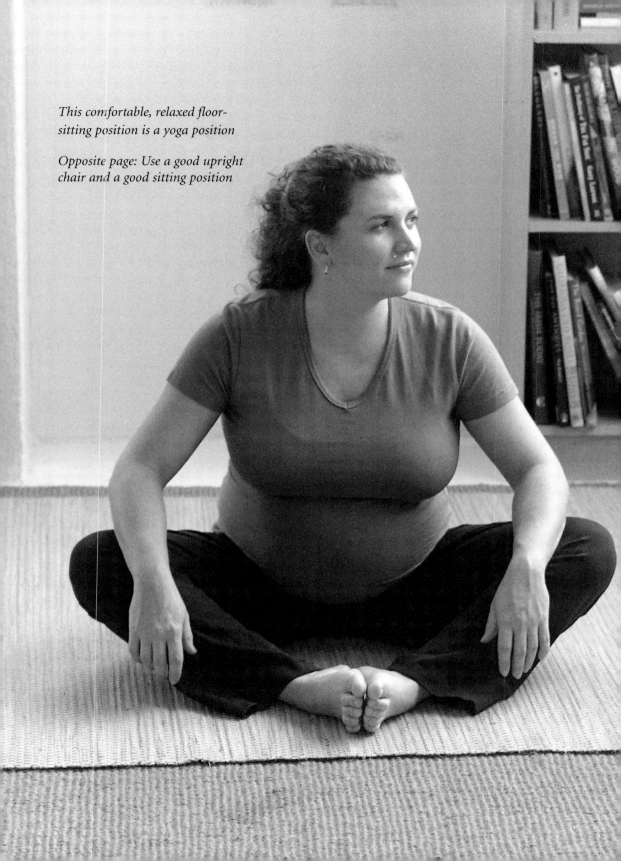

This comfortable, relaxed floor-sitting position is a yoga position

Opposite page: Use a good upright chair and a good sitting position

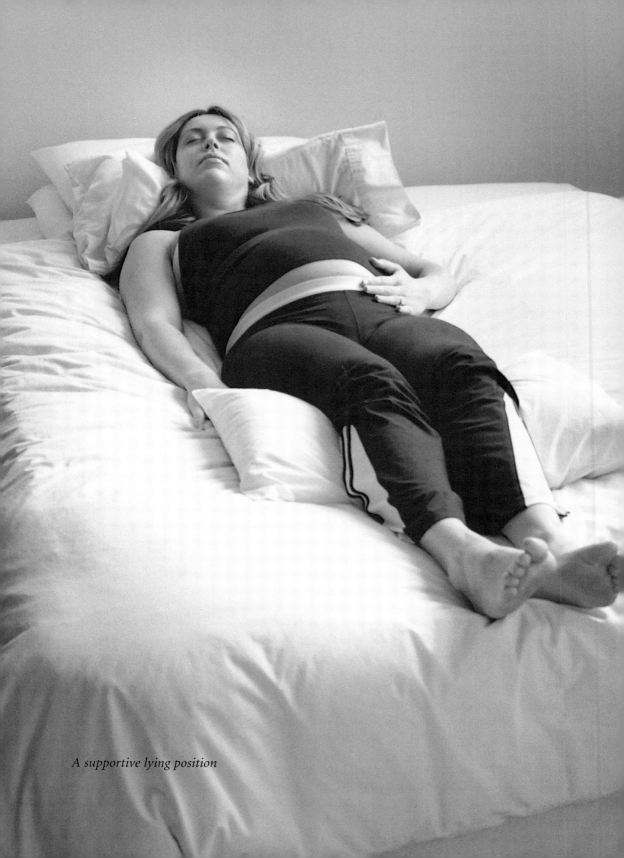

A supportive lying position

lying

What feels right during pregnancy is the most important consideration. Lying on your back, your side or your tummy is a choice that depends on what feels the most comfortable for you – especially considering that lying down, whether it's resting or sleeping, is a major part of your life! There is no right or wrong position; everyone is different. The following text gives you several alternatives.

lying on your back

There are differing opinions about whether or not it is acceptable to lie on your back during pregnancy. Though some health and medical practitioners advise pregnant women not to lie this way, there is no scientific evidence to indicate that this position is harmful to your baby. Be guided by how you feel. If you feel comfortable lying or sleeping on your back, do so. Always check with your doctor or midwife if you are unsure.

If you have always preferred sleeping or resting on your back, try placing a pillow under your knees and a couple of pillows under your head and shoulders. This avoids straining your lower back and it is far more comfortable than lying with your legs out straight. Many pregnant women find this position to be very relaxing and happily sleep cushioned by the pillows. If this position makes you feel a little lightheaded or dizzy, move onto your side or sit up and wait for the dizzy sensation to pass before lying down again.

When you sleep on your back, subconscious mechanisms will cause you to change position if necessary, so there's no need to worry if you fall asleep in this position. Remember, if it feels fine, it usually is.

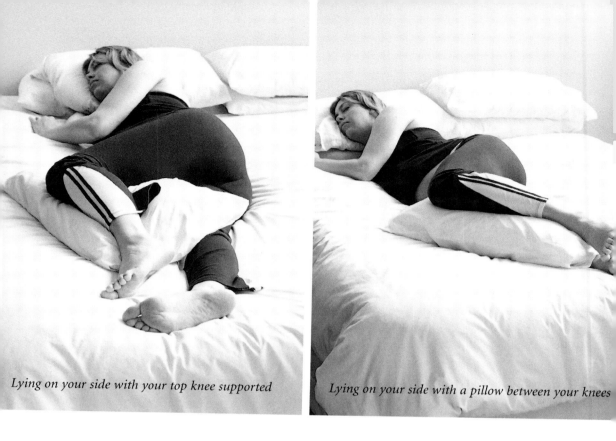

Lying on your side with your top knee supported

Lying on your side with a pillow between your knees

lying on your side

During your pregnancy, the position in which you will probably feel most comfortable for any length of time is lying on your side.

When resting or sleeping on your side, place a pillow between your knees, or rest your top knee on a pillow. This removes the pressure of the upper leg from the lower leg and keeps the hip in a more horizontal position, which reduces the strain on the lower back and hip area. Most pregnant women prefer this very comfortable position, especially during the last few weeks of pregnancy.

lying on your tummy

If you are used to sleeping on your tummy, the good news is that you can still do so in pregnancy. It is important not to lie in this position on a hard surface; you will need a beanbag or pillows for comfort and support.

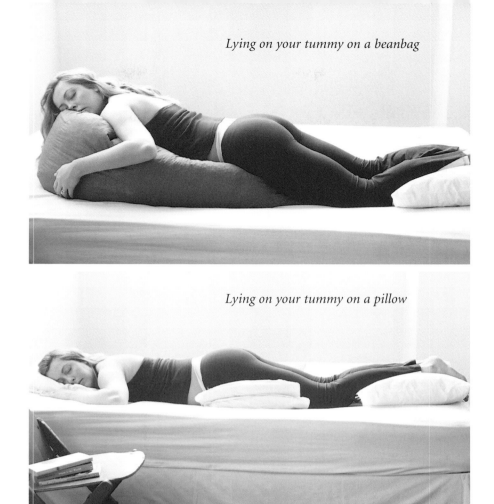

Lying on your tummy on a beanbag

Lying on your tummy on a pillow

If you have a beanbag, place it on the floor or your bed. Punch a large dent in it for your tummy. Lower yourself slowly into the beanbag and place a pillow or two under your feet for comfort. If the discomfort of your increased size prevents you from sleeping well on your back or side, you will welcome this safe, supportive, relaxing position.

If you do not have a beanbag, put pillows under your hips, under your head and shoulders, and under your feet. This is restful for your back and feels wonderful. As always, be guided by how you feel – and never persist in a position that feels uncomfortable or painful.

getting into and out of bed

When pregnant women experience back pain, it can often be related to how they get into and out of bed. Nine times out of ten, they sit on the bed, lower themselves onto their back then lift their legs. To get up, they push themselves up with their arms, then lower their legs to the floor. Wrong! This puts tremendous strain on back and tummy muscles.

The best way to get into bed is to sit on the side of the bed, then lower your body onto your side, while at the same time lifting your legs up, knees bent, keeping your knees together.

To get out of bed, roll onto your side – the side closest to the edge of the bed – then push yourself up, using your arms, lowering your legs at the same time.

Getting into and out of bed from this side-lying position prevents straining your tummy and back muscles because you are not actually using these muscles; the strain is taken by your arms.

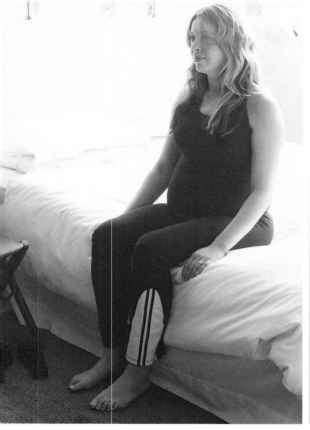
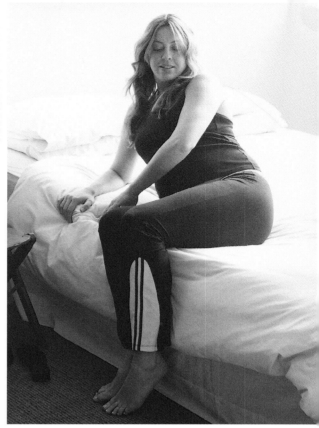

The correct way to get into and out of bed

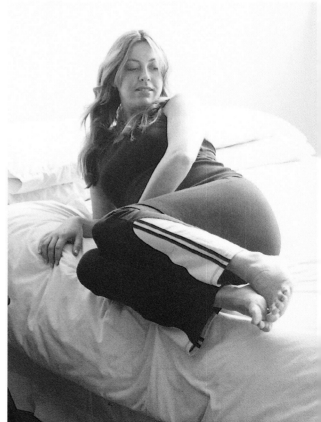

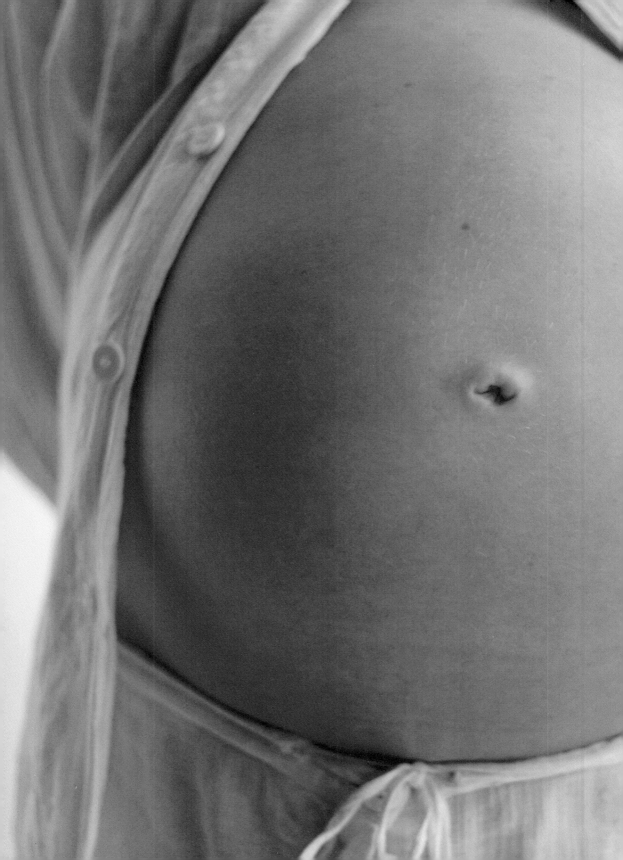

getting into and out of the car

Normally, getting into or out of the car is not something you think about, you just do it, but during pregnancy, with that tummy in front of you, you need to stop and think about this as well as other simple daily movements.

To get into the car, first sit on the car seat with your feet on the ground. Next, support yourself by holding onto the roof and door frames, then lift your feet, either one at a time or together, slowly into the car.

To get out, do the reverse. Turn your body towards the car door, swing your legs out, place your feet on the ground and, using your arms, push your body up and out.

When driving, position your seat so you feel comfortable. Bend your knees slightly, making sure you have enough room to use the pedals without having to straighten your knees fully. You should be sitting with your back in a comfortable position – not too upright, but not set too far back, either. You may like to put a small, soft pillow in the small of your back for added support.

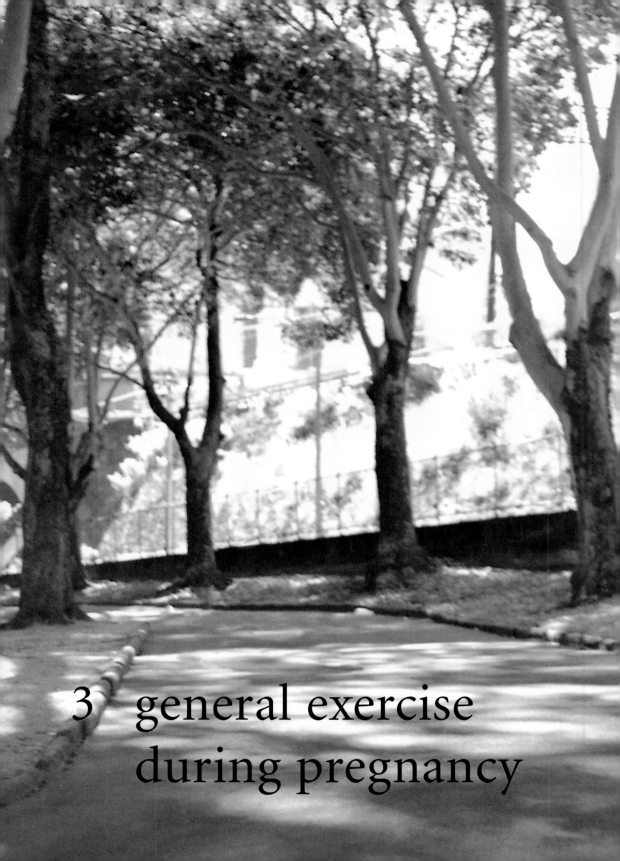

3 general exercise
during pregnancy

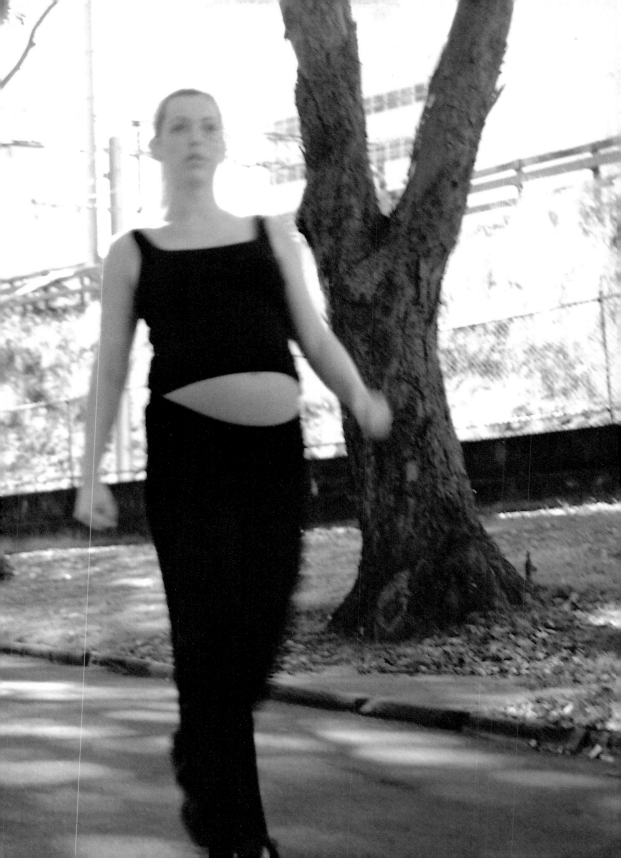

the benefits are clear

You wouldn't dream of going on a 100-kilometre bike ride unless you trained or prepared yourself for it. The same applies to childbirth. Labour means hard work, very hard work! Isn't it sensible, then, to train your body for it by exercising appropriately?

Provided your doctor has given you the all-clear to begin a new exercise program, you should start as soon as possible after your first trimester (12 weeks). Twelve weeks is considered to be the end of the most prolific developmental activity of the embryo, and from around this time the embryo will then be referred to as a foetus. If you have already been exercising regularly, continue to do so, but you may need to modify your routine. If you have been playing high-impact or any type of contact sport, it is preferable to change to low-impact sport and start stretching exercises as well.

There is some controversy surrounding the involvement of pregnant women in contact sport. It is important to bear in mind that any type of contact sport is potentially harmful to your joints, because during pregnancy ligaments become looser, so there is not as much protection for the joints, such as knees, as there would be otherwise. Playing contact sport and the safety considerations for your baby are best discussed with your doctor.

High-impact aerobic exercise is also potentially harmful to your joints and is very taxing on the body during pregnancy, so it is advisable to modify involvement in this type of exercise.

You should be able to take part in whichever form of sensible exercise you choose right up until your baby is born, provided there are no medical reasons recommending against your chosen activity or activities. These are some of the benefits of exercise:

● *Maintains/improves cardiovascular fitness*

Basic exercise such as stationary cycling, walking, swimming or pregnancy fitness classes will make your heart and lungs work harder than activities such as housework or sitting at a desk. Exercising your heart and lungs is highly beneficial, as it enables them to become fitter and thus work more efficiently. As you exercise, your blood circulation speeds up, which brings more vital oxygen to your working muscles.

● *Improves posture and decreases backache*

Regular exercise will strengthen the muscles in your back and improve balance and coordination, which in turn improves posture. As your baby grows, your centre of gravity will alter, which will most likely make you feel a little unbalanced. Modifying your posture will help correct this and avoid possible aches and pains.

● *Strengthens muscles for pregnancy, labour and post-natal recovery*

Regular exercise improves muscle tone and strength, which is beneficial for labour. Also, the fitter you are during pregnancy, the more rapidly you will be able to regain your fitness after delivery.

● *Increases stamina and endurance*

Regular, repetitive exercise will give you the strength and stamina you need – the workout your muscles receive will help them to be much more efficient when called upon during labour. Improving your endurance, the ability to keep going without giving up, through regular exercise will also prepare your muscles for labour – when they need to keep working, without tiring!

● *Maintains/increases flexibility*

The more you exercise, the better your joints and tissues function due to increased blood and oxygen flow. Exercise promotes greater efficiency of movement, less stiffness and fewer aches and pains.

- *Assists in maintenance of healthy weight range*

By exercising and burning calories, the food we eat is used for the body's natural functions – it is not stored as fat. Therefore, during pregnancy, which is usually accompanied by increased appetite, regular exercise helps the extra calories to be distributed effectively.

- *Improves coordination and balance*

As your pregnancy progresses and your body shape and weight change, you will also find that your balance and coordination alter. This is due to the change in your centre of gravity. By exercising regularly, your muscles work to your new shape, which, in turn, feeds back to your brain to enable you to readjust your balance when necessary.

- *Increases feeling of wellbeing and reduces stress and anxiety*

Regular exercise will help you mentally and physically. As you exercise, chemicals secreted by the brain help you to relax and feel good.

when NOT to exercise in pregnancy

- *History of three or more spontaneous miscarriages*

If you have had three or more miscarriages, it may be advisable not to take part in any form of exercise unless your doctor has given you specific approval to do so.

- *Vaginal bleeding or ruptured membranes*

These conditions are best monitored by your doctor and exercise should be avoided, as premature labour is likely.

- *Premature labour*

If labour begins well before your due date, hospitalisation is warranted.

- *Incompetent cervix*

An incompetent cervix is a weakness of the cervix (the neck of the womb) which causes it to open during pregnancy, allowing the amniotic sac to bulge through. This can lead to the sac bursting and abortion of the foetus. If you have this condition and your doctor is aware of it, he or she will usually stitch the cervix to keep it closed. Exercise is best avoided.

● *Placenta praevia*

If your doctor has diagnosed placenta praevia, a condition in which the placenta grows on the lower part of the uterine wall, rather than on the side or at the top, he or she may advise against exercise. The placenta usually moves up as the pregnancy develops, but in some cases it does not. Again, be guided by your doctor.

● *Pregnancy-induced hypertension*

Hypertension is high blood pressure. If a woman becomes hypertensive in pregnancy, it is called pregnancy-induced hypertension. If you have this condition, it will be monitored regularly by your doctor. Exercise should be avoided, as it can cause a further increase in blood pressure.

● *Pre-eclampsia*

This is hypertension plus swelling of the feet, hands and face. It is a serious condition that affects the placenta and reduces the amount of oxygen the baby receives. If you think you might have this condition, see your doctor as soon as possible and avoid exercise.

If you are suffering from any of these conditions, check with your doctor about whether the daily exercises in Chapter 6 are suitable.

exercises recommended for pregnancy

As mentioned above, regular, appropriate exercise will raise your levels of fitness and endurance and increase your ability to cope with labour more effectively. Try to exercise approximately three times a week. If you can't manage this amount of exercise, it is still important to do as much as you can.

On the other hand, pregnancy is not the time to take up exercise such as running or tennis – unless you have been involved in these activities regularly and can continue them at a comfortable level. As discussed on page 28, high-impact sports are not advisable during pregnancy.

The idea of exercise is to feel good. Whenever you are exercising, make sure you are not in any kind of pain. Drink plenty of water and take care not to become overheated. If you feel faint or experience any bleeding, stop immediately.

The following forms of exercise are suitable for pregnant women. They are enjoyable and do not stress the joints or overwork the body. Whichever you choose, try to do it at least three times a week.

WALKING

Walking is the easiest and most convenient form of exercise. It has an aerobic component, working your heart and lungs; and a strengthening component, toning the muscles in your bottom and legs. If you are not fit to start with, begin walking short distances and increase the distance over time. It is not necessary to build up a sweat; use your common sense and stop when you feel you have had enough. Steady walking for approximately 30 minutes is usually sufficient to begin with.

SWIMMING

Swimming is an excellent form of exercise during pregnancy, as the water buoys you up and makes you feel almost weightless. As with walking, swim as far as you like and for as long as it feels good. Always start swimming a short distance and increase it over time. Swimming is a great aerobic workout – exercising your heart and lungs – as well as toning your arm, leg and back muscles.

CYCLING

Cycling is a highly beneficial form of exercise during pregnancy, especially if it is already part of your fitness regime. It is preferable to use a stationary exercise bike rather than a pushbike during your pregnancy, to avoid the risk of falling and potentially harming yourself or your baby. As with any other form of exercise, start with a short stint, then build up your exercise periods as your fitness level increases. Work within your comfort range and never exercise against a high resistance. You do not have to work up a sweat to benefit from this exercise, nor should you exercise until you are breathless.

FITNESS CLASSES

Not all fitness classes will suit you while you are pregnant. Regular gym fitness classes are not the best form of exercise, as you will need to avoid some of the exercises. It is best to attend a specialised pregnancy fitness class if at all possible. Some maternity hospitals run these types of classes.

If these are not available in your area, opt for low-impact fitness classes or stretch classes, but check with the instructor before you start to ensure that he or she is aware that you are pregnant and should not be performing some of the exercises.

Avoid high-impact exercises, as they can strain your softened ligaments and joints.

YOGA

Yoga is one of the best forms of exercise for stretching and relaxing. Again, it is advisable to find a specialised pregnancy class, or make sure the yoga instructor is aware of your pregnancy.

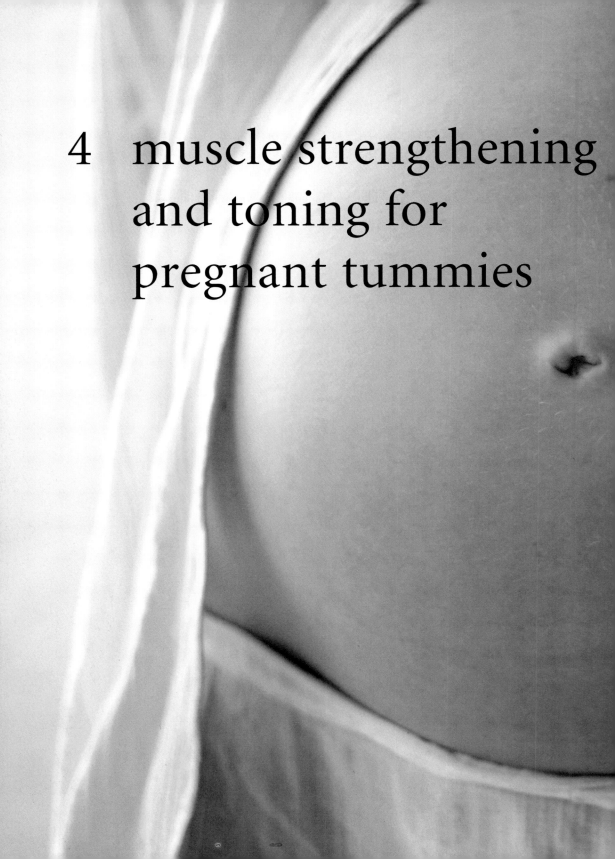

4 muscle strengthening and toning for pregnant tummies

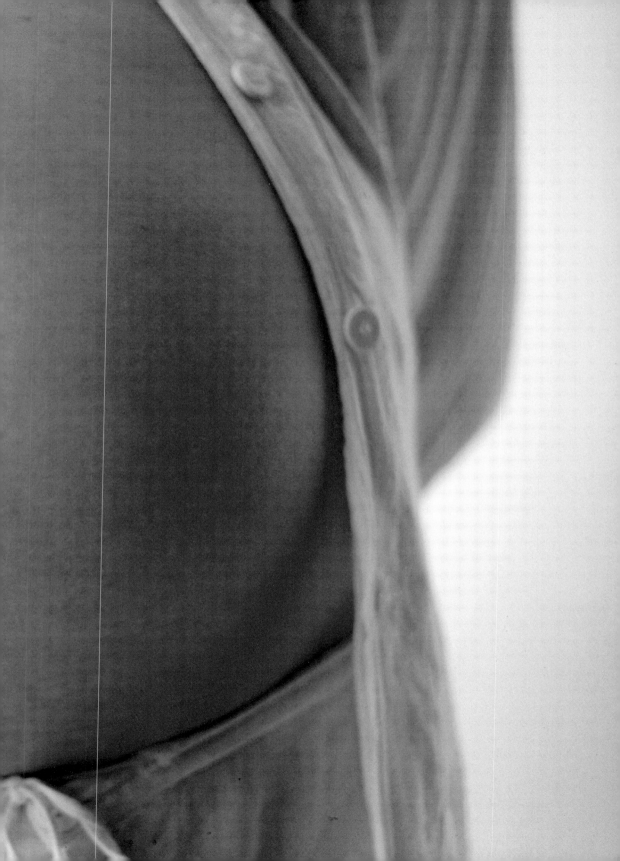

abdominal muscle separation

We have just seen how important it is to exercise regularly in preparation for childbirth to build up fitness and endurance levels, but there are also specific muscle groups that require special attention during pregnancy. These are your abdominal muscles and your leg and thigh muscles.

During pregnancy, your longitudinal abdominal muscles come apart, or separate, to some extent (see diagrams opposite). This separation is normal and the size of the separation differs from woman to woman.

You can feel for this separation when you lie on your back and lift your head – a 'popping out' area may appear down the middle of your tummy. This indicates where the abdominal muscles are separating. You can also see the separation when you lean backwards.

The average abdominal muscle separation in a woman who is pregnant for the first time is approximately one to two finger-widths. It is relatively easy to reduce this kind of muscle separation after childbirth.

Women who have poor muscle tone, who have had more than one pregnancy, and have not exercised or strengthened their tummy muscles, may have a larger separation of approximately three or more finger-widths. A larger separation means less support for the growing uterus and a much greater strain on the back muscles. Without appropriate abdominal strengthening exercises, this separation may reduce a little after birth, but not significantly, and could lead to long-term back problems.

Therefore, it is important that a physiotherapist or midwife check your abdominal muscle separation after you give birth. You should then be monitored regularly until the separation is down to one finger-width.

If, when leaving hospital, the separation is over three finger-widths, you should wear a binder to support your back and tummy until the separation decreases. This would be supplied by the hospital.

BEFORE PREGNANCY

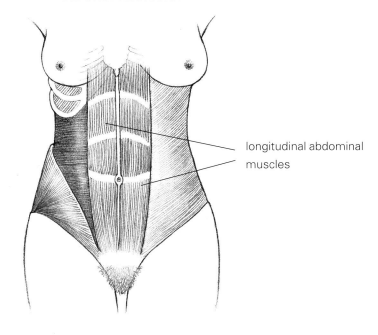

longitudinal abdominal
muscles

DURING PREGNANCY

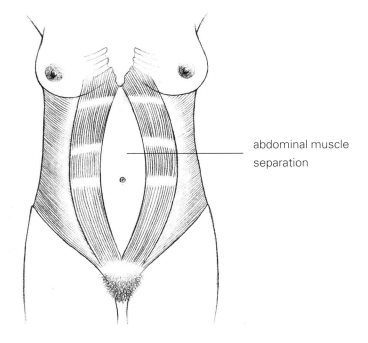

abdominal muscle
separation

muscle strengthening and toning for pregnant tummies 37

case study

problem: At 23 weeks, Sophie, complained of feeling fat and having a strange 'tearing' sensation in her tummy muscles. She said it felt like the muscles were ripping, especially when she was moving around in bed or getting into and out of the car.

cause: Sophie had a smallish separation of her abdominal muscles. With her slim build, as her uterus grew larger, it was pushing on and stretching her abdominal muscles, creating the discomfort she was complaining of.

treatment: Sophie massaged her tummy daily with pure sweet almond oil and regularly practised simple abdominal exercises, such as pulling her tummy muscles in, holding for one breath in and out, then releasing them. She repeated these in sets of five as often as she could throughout the day. These simple exercises helped strengthen her tummy muscles, and the massage helped soften and relax them. I also reminded her that she was pregnant, not fat!

abdominal exercises

All you need to do to tone your abdominal muscles during pregnancy is simply contract and tighten them. Whether you are standing, sitting or lying, just pull your tummy muscles in, hold them tightly for approximately 5 seconds, then relax them. Repeat in sets of five as often as you can during the day. Try not to hold your breath while you tighten the muscles. Perform this safe, simple, effective tightening exercise at any stage during your pregnancy.

Practising this exercise to keep your abdominal muscles toned will help you recover your 'normal' tummy shape more quickly after childbirth. If you have been used to doing sit-up exercises prior to your pregnancy, continue doing them, provided there are no medical reasons why you should not. Check with your midwife or doctor. Obviously, it is not advisable to do 100 sit-ups a day – approximately five to ten a day is adequate. Note: Never sit up directly from lying. Lift only your head and shoulders and keep your knees bent.

The gentle exercises on the next two pages will also help you tone and strengthen your abdominal area. Check with a physiotherapist if you are not sure how to do them correctly.

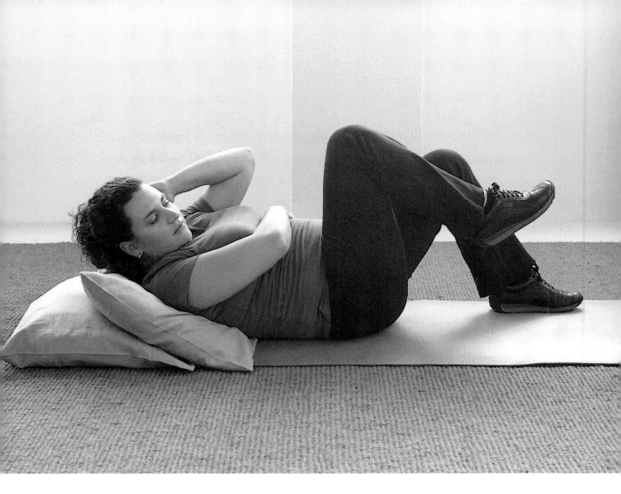

Half sit-up

1 Lie on your back with your knees bent and your feet on the floor, shoulder-width apart.

2 Place your left hand behind your head.

3 Gently supporting your left side with your right hand, lift your right knee slightly and bring your left elbow towards the knee (they shouldn't touch). Hold for 3 seconds, then relax.

Repeat on the other side. Three to five repetitions on each side once a day is sufficient. Try not to hold your breath.

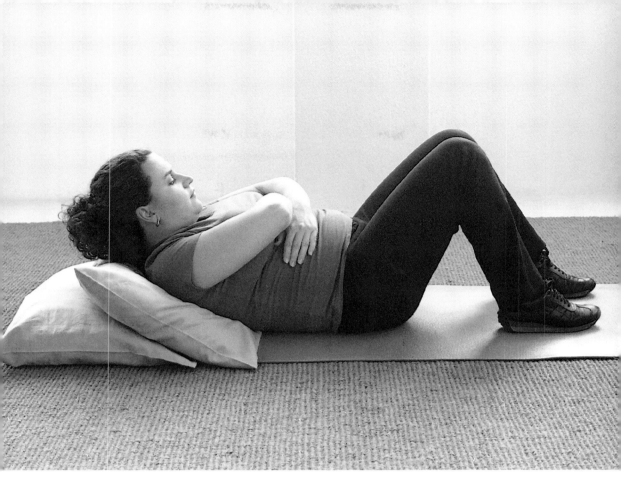

Head and shoulder lift

1 Lie on your back with your knees bent and your feet on the floor, shoulder-width apart.

2 Tighten your abdominal muscles and lift your head and shoulders off the floor, keeping your lower back flat on the floor. (Do not do a straight sit-up.)

Hold for 3–5 seconds, then relax and come down.

Repeat five times slowly. Stop if you feel dizzy or nauseous.

Do not hold your breath.

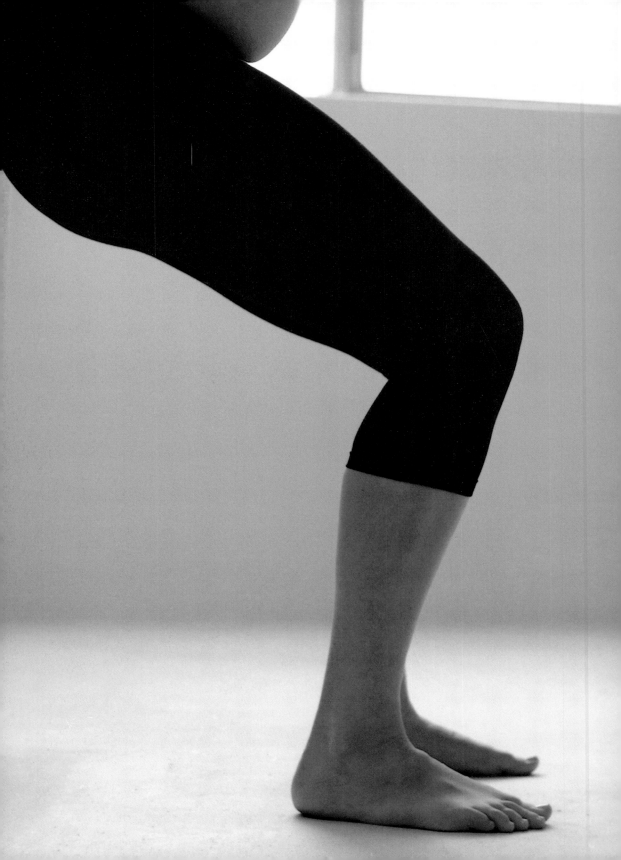

5 muscle strengthening for legs and thighs

leg and thigh muscles

The aims of exercising in pregnancy are to improve muscle tone and cardio-vascular fitness and to increase flexibility, but specific strengthening exercises for your legs and thighs can be highly beneficial too. Exercising these muscles aids blood circulation in the lower limbs, which helps to decrease swelling in the feet and legs and reduce muscle cramps.

It's about preparing for labour as well. The stronger your quadriceps muscles (the muscles at the front of the upper legs), the longer you will be able to hold certain positions during labour; the greater your strength, stamina and endurance, the more control you will have over your body; and the more cardiovascular exercise you do during pregnancy, ie walking, cycling or swimming, the greater your endurance will be.

leg and thigh exercises

One of the best leg and thigh toning exercises is walking. Yes, walking. Head out for a 30-minute walk at least three times a week and you will be on the way to strong legs and thighs. If you live near the beach, walking in soft sand is particularly effective as it gives added resistance to your leg muscles. Cycling on a stationary bike or walking on a treadmill are also beneficial, but always use a low resistance level.

Another easy exercise is walking in the water in a swimming pool. The resistance of water will help tone and strengthen your leg muscles and give you some cardiovascular exercise too. To do it effectively, walk the length of a 25-metre pool at least five times. Build up to this if you did not do any exercise prior to your pregnancy.

If you really want to challenge yourself and tone these muscles, the wall squat exercise opposite (illustrated over) is highly beneficial. It is neither easy nor pleasant, but it will demonstrate to you, to a certain extent, what your reaction might be when you experience painful muscle contractions as you will during labour. Try it with your partner and observe his reaction!

You can also establish what your coping techniques might be during labour, whether it is massaging the aching muscles, using breathing techniques, or visualisation, or other relaxation or releasing methods, such as yelling or screaming – whatever works for you. And as you test yourself with this exercise, you will be strengthening your leg muscles all the while. Walk around a bit after doing this exercise to help ease those sore quadriceps muscles.

Wall squats

1 Stand with your back against a wall, your feet shoulder-width apart.

2 Tilt your pelvis so that your back is flat against the wall, then slide down to a half-squatting position (see the photo over). Hold that position. After 5–10 seconds, you will feel your leg muscles (quads) contracting and hurting. This discomfort will increase as you continue to hold the position. Try to hold it for 60 seconds, which is the average length of a contraction in labour.

3 Straighten up, shake your legs, and repeat once more, if you dare! Try to do this exercise at least four to six times a week.

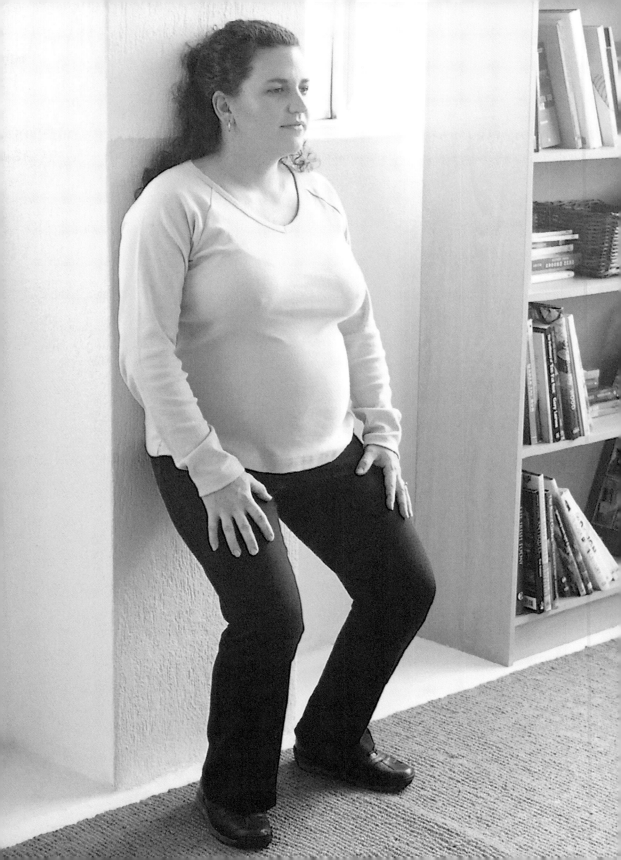

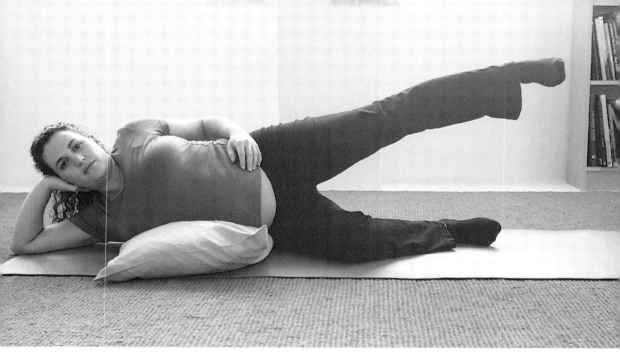

Leg lifts

Leg lifts are leg-toning exercises you can do lying on your side, on the floor or the bed. Start by doing ten repetitions per day on each side, and build up the number gradually. To make the exercise more challenging, attach a Velcro leg weight to your ankle.

Leg lifts

1 Lying on your side, bend the lower leg and keep it firmly on the floor.
2 Slowly lift the top leg, keeping it straight, foot flexed, not pointed.
3 Lower it slowly and lift again.
Repeat ten times, then change to the other side. Note: When changing sides, roll slowly from one side to the other.

The wall squat – a quads-strengthening exercise

6 key daily exercises

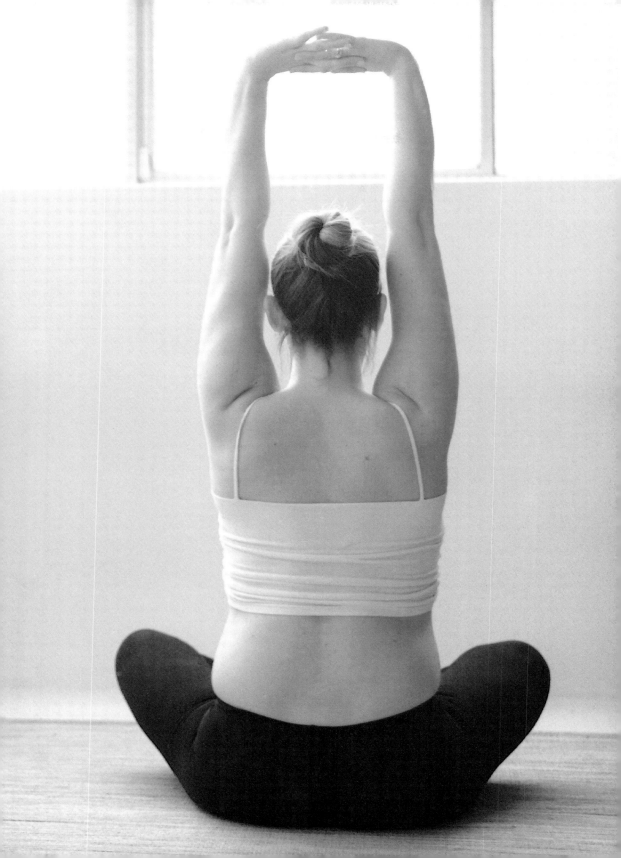

back

If you spend long hours sitting at a computer or working with your hands, the following upper back exercises will help relieve tight, sore muscles between your shoulder blades and between your neck and shoulders. Practise these simple, effective exercises as often as you can.

Shoulder circles
1 Place your hands on your shoulders.
2 Circle your elbows up towards your ears, then back, in big, slow circling movements. Always circle backwards, as if swimming backstroke.
Repeat six times, then follow with the upper back stretch.

Upper back stretch
1 Clasp your hands behind your back and pull your arms straight.
Hold for 5 seconds, then release.
Repeat twice, then do two or three more shoulder circles.

If practised daily, the following spinal stretches will help keep your back supple and release tightness or strain. The bridging exercise will help strengthen your lower back and buttocks – it is even said to help turn a breech baby. These exercises are best done on the floor.
Always perform these exercises slowly and if you experience cramping or pain, stop until the pain subsides. Remember to breathe normally, and never hold your breath.

Half spinal stretch
1 Lie on your back, with your arms out, knees bent and feet on the floor.
2 Tilt your pelvis so that your lower back flattens against the floor.

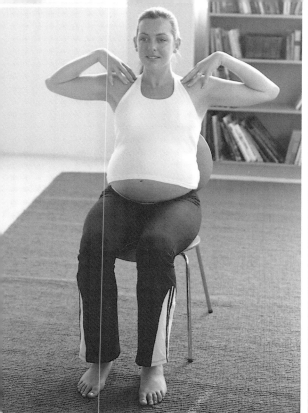

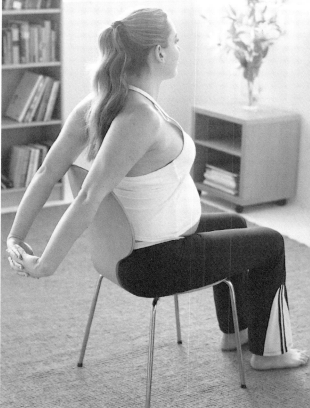

Shoulder circles *Upper back stretch*

3 Keeping them together, turn your knees to one side as far as you can without lifting the opposite shoulder. Make sure your head is facing in the opposite direction to your knees. Hold for 5 seconds, then slowly roll to the other side. Do three stretches on each side, slowly!

Full spinal stretch

1 Lie on your back with your arms stretched out to the sides.

2 Stretch out your left leg. Hook your right foot under your left knee, then roll your right knee to the left over your body, until you feel your right shoulder beginning to lift. Stop there, making sure that your shoulders are flat on the ground.

3 With your head turned to the right, hold for 10 seconds, then change to the other side. Do two to three stretches on each side.

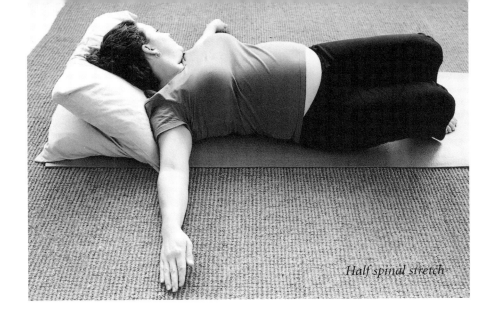

Half spinal stretch

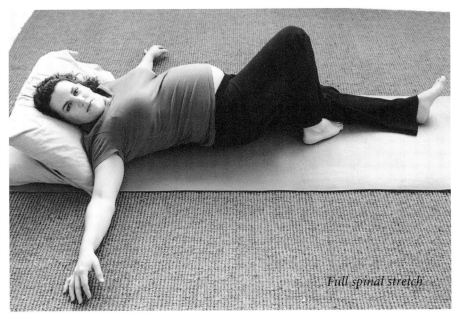

Full spinal stretch

Bridging exercise

1 Lie on your back, your knees comfortably apart and feet on the floor.

2 Slowly lift your bottom (not too high – don't arch your lower back).

3 Squeeze your buttocks together, count to five, then slowly lower
yourself down, relaxing your buttocks. Repeat three times.

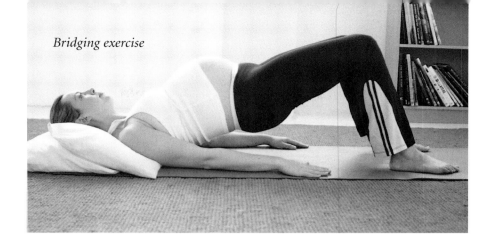

Bridging exercise

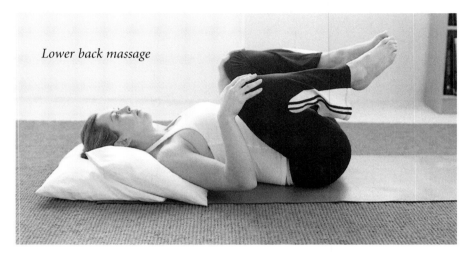

Lower back massage

Lower back massage and pelvic mobiliser

1 Lying on your back, bring your knees to your chest one at a time.

2 Place your hands on your knees, keeping your knees apart.

3 Slowly roll your lower back in a circle against the floor.

Do six circles in one direction, then six in the other.

The key to doing these exercises effectively is to do them slowly.
Doing them too quickly will prevent the muscles from stretching
properly and can even cause a 'stitch' in the groin.

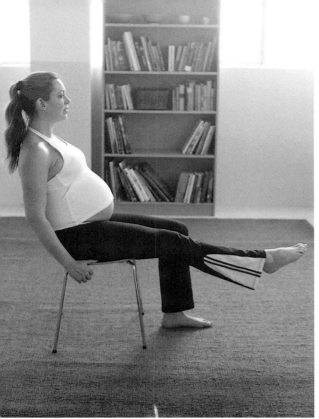
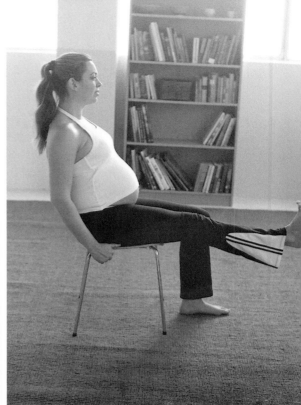

Pointing and flexing the feet

legs and feet

When you have been sitting for a while, or whenever you feel the need, stretch your legs out straight, then bring your toes up towards you. Hold in this flexed position for a few seconds, then point your toes; flex and point several times, either both feet together or separately.

Do this as often as you can throughout the day and also before you go to sleep at night. It will decrease the incidence of cramping.

Elevating your legs and feet will also help decrease swelling and aid circulation. Always make sure that your feet are higher than your heart. Pointing and flexing your feet in this position is beneficial. Do this on the floor with your legs up against the wall, or when you're lying in bed.

pelvis

Running from the pubic bone at the front of the body to the coccyx bone at the back, the muscles of the pelvic floor surround the anus, vagina and urethra and also support the pelvic organs, such as the bladder, the uterus and the bowel. These muscles aren't visible externally, but you can feel them when you consciously contract them.

During pregnancy, your muscles and ligaments soften due to the hormonal changes taking place in your body. This is entirely normal. However, this softening effect, combined with the pressure the growing uterus exerts on the pelvic floor muscles, not to mention that of the baby moving through this area during a vaginal delivery, can all cause weakening and stretching. Therefore, it is extremely important to exercise these muscles regularly – if you don't, the likelihood of suffering from problems such as incontinence or prolapse later in life increases. The higher the number of vaginal deliveries you have in your lifetime, the greater the chance of these problems occurring.

PELVIC FLOOR CROSS-SECTION   PELVIC FLOOR CROSS-SECTION WITH PROLAPSE

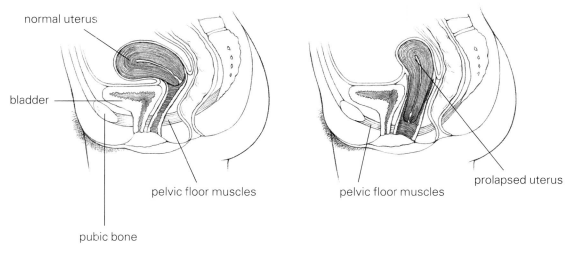

normal uterus

bladder

pelvic floor muscles

pubic bone

pelvic floor muscles

prolapsed uterus

NORMAL POSITION OF PELVIC FLOOR MUSCLES

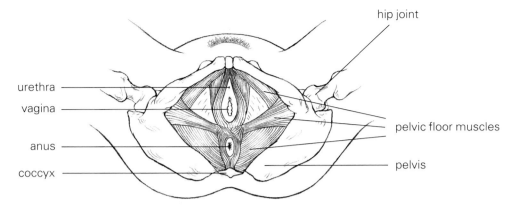

hip joint

urethra

vagina

anus

coccyx

pelvic floor muscles

pelvis

POSITION OF PELVIC FLOOR MUSCLES DURING VAGINAL DELIVERY

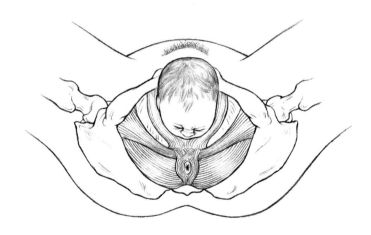

PELVIS BONES

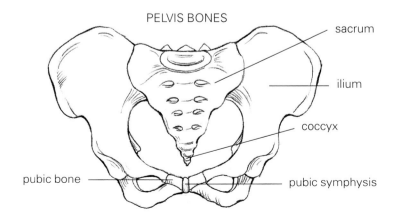

sacrum

ilium

coccyx

pubic bone

pubic symphysis

Incontinence is the loss of urine when running, jumping, sneezing or coughing. Another sign of incontinence is being unable to 'hold on', and not making it to the toilet in time. Don't panic if you experience this in the later stages of pregnancy – it is quite normal. However, it should not persist after your baby is born.

As women approach and enter menopause, they undergo major hormonal changes. The levels of oestrogen and progesterone in the body decrease, causing connective tissue, ligaments and muscles to soften, and this includes the pelvic floor muscles. If a woman does not exercise to keep these muscles toned during her younger years, once menopause comes around, these muscles will weaken further. The insufficient support for the uterus, bladder and bowel can lead to incontinence problems and sometimes prolapse – the 'dropping down' of the uterus or bladder.

So, it is vitally important to exercise your pelvic floor muscles as often as possible throughout and after your pregnancy to maintain their tone. It is recommended that you keep on exercising right up until your baby is born, then recommence the exercises after a rest period of 24 hours.

Incontinence or prolapse is a common problem later in life and many women see it as an inevitable part of ageing – it is not, and no woman should have to put up with it. There is help available – if you think you may have incontinence or prolapse problems, mention it to your doctor, who will refer you to a specialist physiotherapist, continence advisor or specialist doctor.

pelvic floor exercises

Whenever you stop the flow of urine mid-flow, you are using your pelvic floor muscles. When you next need to empty your bladder, try this: Sit on the toilet, start the flow of urine, then after a couple of moments, before your bladder is empty, stop the flow. Let out a little bit, stop again, then empty your bladder completely.

Did you feel the muscles tightening? Could you stop the flow? If you did, your pelvic floor muscles are in good shape. If not, start exercising! (Note: It is not advisable to try to stop the flow of urine every time you go to the toilet, as it can lead to bladder problems.)

Pelvic floor exercises should be a part of your daily life. Try to associate a daily activity with doing them, for example, every time you have something to drink, or stop at a red traffic light, do the exercises. You will find them easy to do once you become familiar with them – the difficulty will be in remembering to do them. And the more exercises you do, the better, but it is best to do them in groups of five to ten.

Do these exercises on a daily basis and continue for the rest of your life! If you find that despite regularly exercising your pelvic floor muscles you still have incontinence problems, see your doctor.

QUICK CONTRACTIONS

Wherever you are, whether you're sitting, standing or lying, you can exercise your pelvic floor muscles. Simply squeeze the muscles tightly, hold for a moment, then release them. Try five to ten of these contractions at a time, as often as you can throughout the day.

SLOW CONTRACTIONS

Another exercise you can practise at any time of the day, in any position, is the slow pelvic floor contraction.

Squeeze your pelvic floor muscles tightly, then pull them up towards your belly-button. Without holding your breath, hold the position for the count of five, then release gently. Start doing three to five of these at a time, then, as your muscles strengthen, build up to ten in a row.

PELVIC TILTING

Pelvic tilting is a simple and effective exercise for reducing lower back-ache due to stiffness or poor posture. It is not only beneficial during pregnancy, but can be done at any time, in any place and in virtually any position. While pelvic tilting may take some practice, once you can do it correctly, it should be relaxing and soothing, helping to release a tight, tense lower back.

You may like to do these pelvic tilts in front of a mirror so that you can see if you are arching and releasing your lower back correctly. Kneeling is the easiest position for the pelvic tilt and you get a greater range of movement in this position – it feels great!

When you are working at a desk or sitting for long periods of time, try a few pelvic tilts every now and then without stopping what you are doing. This will prevent your lower back from tightening and aching. If your workmates look at you strangely, explain the exercise to them.

When standing for long periods, in a queue or at the stove, do a few pelvic tilts in that position to achieve the same effect. You don't have to be pregnant to benefit from this simple exercise, either.

Pelvic tilt, sitting

1 Sit on a hard-backed, supportive chair (not a sofa) with your arms relaxed and feet comfortably on the floor.
2 Move your hip bones forward then backward, rocking slowly and smoothly. Try not to lean your body forward or backward, and keep your shoulders still. Try not to jerk, just rock slowly

Pelvic tilt, standing

1 Stand with your feet comfortably apart, your hands on your hips and your knees slightly bent.

2 Slowly tilt your pelvis forward and back five to ten times.

Pelvic tilt, lying

1 Lie on the floor (not on the bed or sofa) with your knees bent, feet comfortably apart and arms comfortable.

2 Tilt your pelvis so you feel your lower back flatten against the floor, then tilt away from the floor. Repeat five to ten times, slowly.

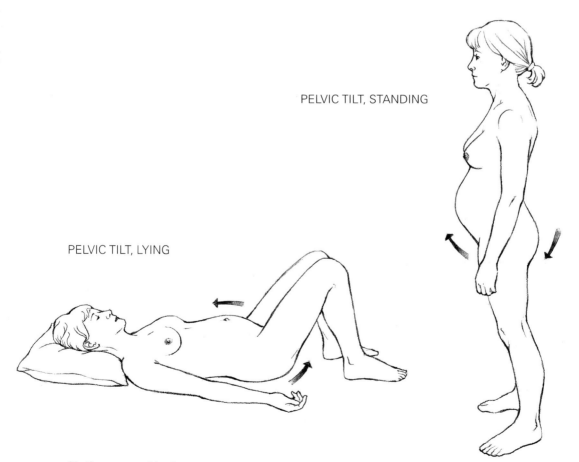

PELVIC TILT, STANDING

PELVIC TILT, LYING

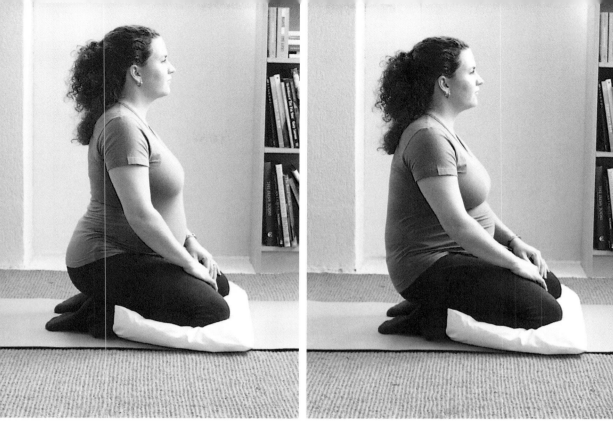

Pelvic tilt, kneeling

Pelvic tilt, kneeling

1 Kneel on your bed or on a pillow on the floor.

2 Tilt your pelvis backward and forward in a slow, rocking motion.
Repeat five to ten times.

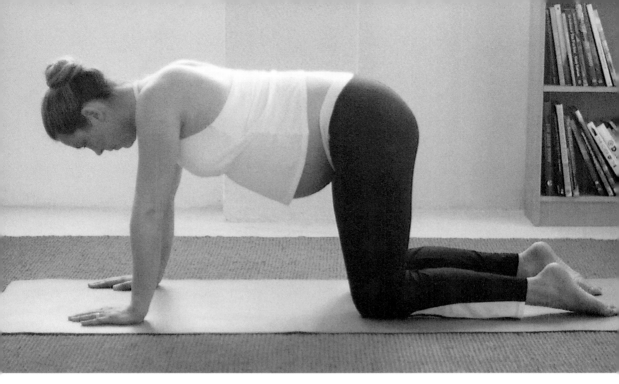

Pelvic belly dancing

pelvic belly dancing

Pelvic belly dancing is an excellent releasing exercise for your back, tummy and pelvic area. It is a lovely, relaxing, easy movement that also releases tight muscles and takes pressure off your back. You can do it any time during your pregnancy and as often as you like.

In fact, do it as often as you can. If you can't manage it during the day, try to do this exercise in the evening before you go to sleep. This will relax your muscles and help you sleep. If you wake during the night due to discomfort, do a few pelvic circles slowly, then try to sleep again once you have relaxed.

During labour, many women do pelvic belly dancing on all fours to help reduce back pain caused by the baby lying in the posterior position (ie with the baby's spine sitting against the mother's spine, causing pressure that leads to back pain). Your midwife will guide and advise you at the appropriate time for this exercise if this is the case.

Standing

1 Stand with your feet shoulder-width apart, your knees slightly bent and your hands on your hips.

2 Circle your pelvis slowly in one direction six times, then change and circle in the other direction. You can do this exercise in labour, either between contractions to relax the pelvic area, or during contractions if you feel you need to move.

Kneeling

1 Kneel on all fours on the floor or bed. Your knees and arms should be shoulder-width apart.

2 Circle your pelvis slowly six times in one direction then change and circle in the other direction. Try to keep the movements in the horizontal plane, not up and down or side to side. Just imagine you are drawing big circles with your bottom.

the yoga stretch

The yoga stretch is another very comfortable and relaxing position. It stretches the back muscles, easing tension along the spine and also helps to stretch the inner thighs, hips, lower and upper back, and helps to open out the pelvic area in preparation for labour. You should try to start doing this stretch as early in your pregnancy as possible, continuing throughout your pregnancy. It's also highly beneficial to start practising it again in the post-natal period as soon as you can and continue for as long as you feel the benefits.

It is important to note that sitting in a sofa or a chair when you are relaxing will do nothing constructive for your back muscles – nothing to

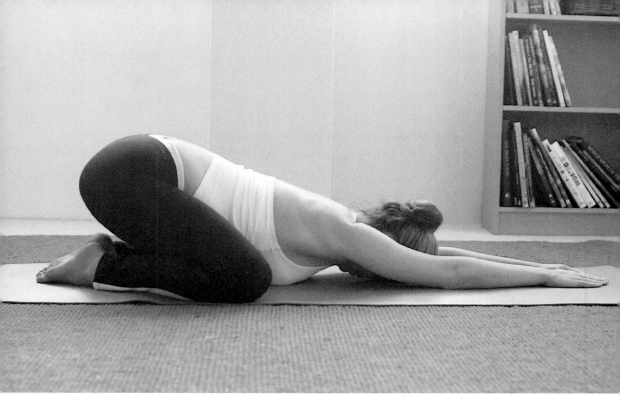

Full yoga stretch

prepare your body for labour – so whenever possible, get down into the yoga stretch position to read, to watch television or just to relax. This position is said to encourage the baby to lie in the anterior position within the uterus (ie the baby lies with his or her back to the front or to the side of the uterus). The anterior position, rather than the posterior position, is the one favoured for a smoother delivery.

You can perform the yoga stretch on the floor or on your bed, which-ever you prefer, and, like pelvic belly dancing, it's an exercise you should do as often as possible.

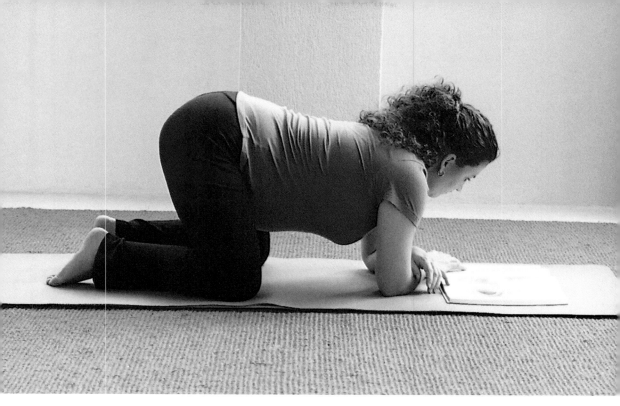

Half yoga stretch – a comfortable position for reading

Yoga stretch

Kneeling, keeping your feet together and your knees shoulder-width apart, stretch forward with your arms straight out in front of you and your head down. Try to position your bottom as close to your feet as possible. If this feels awkward, bend your elbows and place your forehead on your hands.

Hold the stretch for approximately 2 minutes, and build up to 20 minutes as it becomes easier over time. If you find your growing tummy is uncomfortable in this position, just raise your bottom.

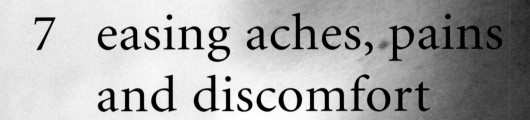

7 easing aches, pains and discomfort

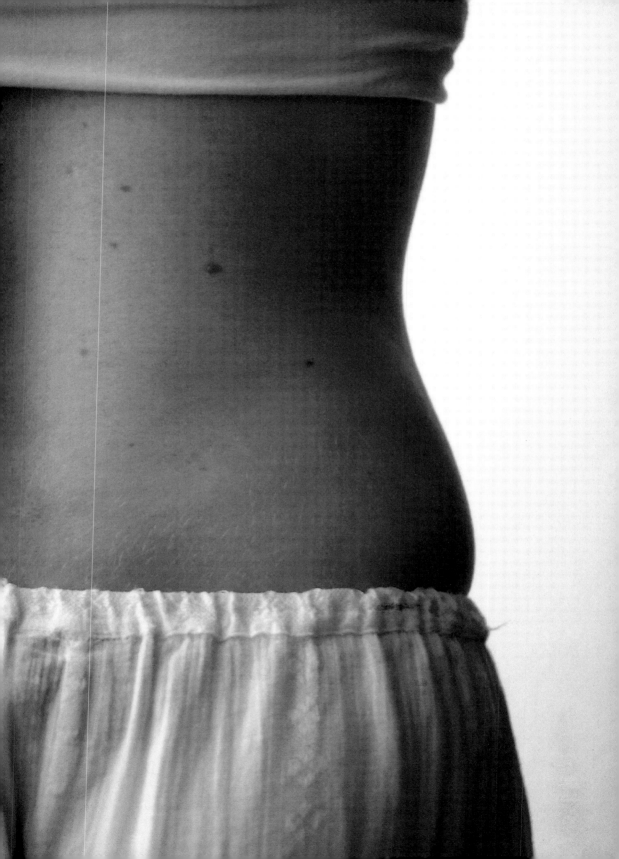

tiredness

Feeling tired and having less energy than you had before you were pregnant is quite normal, and to be expected, especially during the first trimester (12 weeks), and also towards the end of the last trimester.

Whenever you wonder why you are feeling so listless, think of all that extra weight you are carrying around, as well as the many other body changes you are coping with. Your body is doing a remarkable job.

easing the tiredness

Whenever possible, try to spend at least half an hour, preferably in the afternoon, lying down, with your legs elevated to reduce any swelling or aching. Have a nap or simply relax. This will help restore energy.

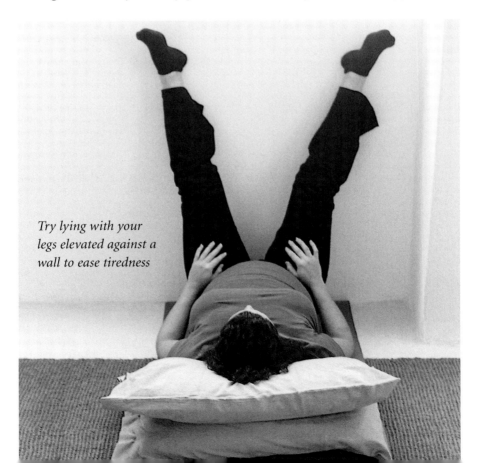

Try lying with your legs elevated against a wall to ease tiredness

Exercise will help improve circulation, get your muscles moving and your heart pumping, and it is enjoyable too. Go for a swim, a walk, or attend yoga or fitness classes designed for pregnant women; basic exercise will refresh you and increase your fitness, endurance and energy levels.

If you are exercising regularly, but still feel listless or lacking in energy, see your doctor for a check-up. Ensure that your diet is providing you with all the vitamins and minerals you and your growing baby need.

upper back pain

This is pain felt either between the shoulder blades, across the shoulder blades, or between the neck and shoulder. It can be caused by a change in posture due to enlarged breasts and upper back stooping or sitting at a desk or computer for long periods without stretching, so that the upper back and neck muscles tire. This pain is usually worse at the end of the day. When sitting at a desk or computer, ensure that you are sitting square, not slightly rotated, as this will cause one-sided upper back pain.

easing the pain

It is important to stop what you are doing every hour or so and do some shoulder circles (see page 50).

If you feel a 'knot' or a painful area between your shoulder blades, try a few upper back stretches (see page 50). Follow this with a few vertical shoulder stretches.

Vertical shoulder stretch
1 Sitting or standing, stretch your arms straight up as far as you can.
2 Hold for 5 seconds, then relax and bring your arms down.

lower back pain

Lower back pain is the most common complaint during pregnancy; and different women experience it in different ways.

Lower back pain during pregnancy is due to the hormone-related softening of the ligaments around the pelvis and lower back in preparation for childbirth, and to the resultant postural changes. This softening, along with the extra weight of the growing uterus and your constantly changing centre of gravity, leads to lower back pain which you might feel either right across your lower back, or only on one side. It may even radiate down one or both legs. All of these experiences are quite normal in pregnancy. These pains, once assessed accurately, can be managed well with the correct advice and patient cooperation.

More often than not, sitting, bending or lifting incorrectly contributes further to lower back pain. This is when you can take care to minimise it. Another major cause of lower back pain is getting in and out of bed incorrectly.

easing the pain

When you're doing household chores such as ironing, vacuuming and hanging out washing, make sure that you keep your back straight. When you bend, use your knees, not your back. Ensure the ironing board is at waist-height. Don't lift anything heavy – ask someone to help you – and perhaps use a trolley for your washing basket to avoid lifting heavy, wet washing. When doing activities such as sweeping or vacuuming, try to lunge rather than twisting your body. An upright vacuum cleaner is preferable to a pull-along barrel type.

When at work, if you tend to sit most of the time, ensure that you have a good, supportive chair. Keep your back straight, and put your feet

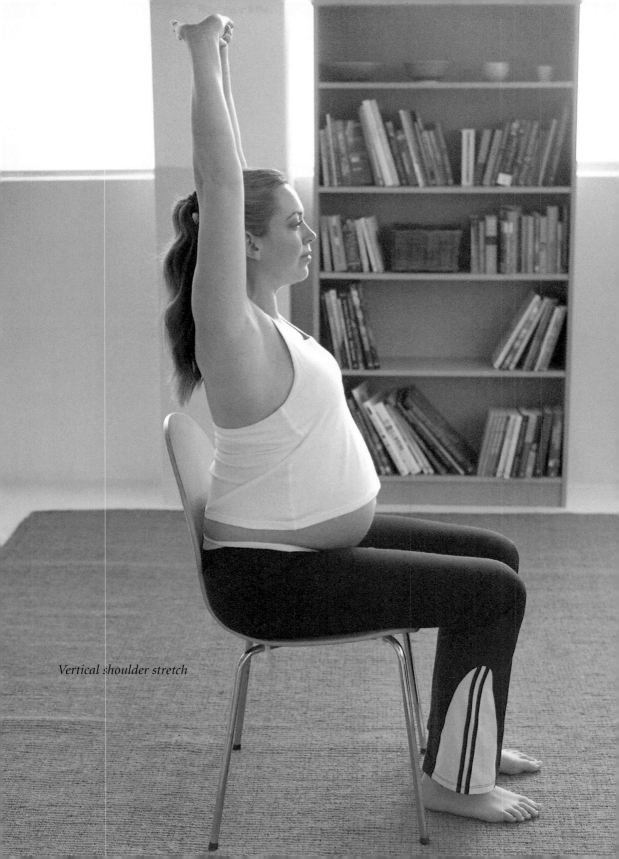

Vertical shoulder stretch

on a foot stool or a couple of telephone books if possible. If using a zcomputer, position it so it is directly in front of you, not off to one side, as this can lead to one-sided lower and upper back and neck stiffness.

If you stand most of the day as part of your job, try to do a few pelvic tilts and shoulder circles every couple of hours (see page 50). When possible, wear supportive, comfortable shoes with an arch support and a low heel. Unsupportive shoes can be one of the causes of lower backache. Have your feet checked by a podiatrist, as you may benefit from having arch supports.

The golden rule is: always keep your back straight. The more you are aware of your posture, the easier it will become, and the less likelihood of straining your back. Here are some further suggestions for avoiding lower back pain:

● Try getting used to the squatting position, since this may be beneficial for labour. Whenever you pick something up or put something down, whether it is light or heavy, bend your knees, not your back.

● When a toddler wants to be picked up, entice him or her onto a chair so that you will not have to bend down too far.

● When getting out of bed, make sure that you roll onto your side first. Never pull yourself up into a sitting position (see page 22). This will ensure that you don't strain your back or tummy muscles.

If, however, you follow these simple rules and find that your backache persists or worsens with time, contact your doctor or a pregnancy physiotherapist. Any of the women's hospitals or the Australian Physiotherapy Association will be able to advise you on how to contact one of these specialists (see Resources, page 126).

case study

problem: Susie complained of a sore, tight lower back. She was 18 weeks pregnant with her first child and said the pain was bearable, but annoying and a little worrying. She was experiencing quite a bad ache whenever she sat for a while, or when she got up after sitting. Once she began moving, the pain eased slightly.

cause: This is a very common complaint. In early pregnancy, there is a lot of softening taking place around the pelvis due to hormonal changes. The body's centre of gravity is changing, and the softened ligaments and muscles create a less stable lower back and pelvic area.

treatment: Posture is all-important! When Susie was relaxing on her sofa, she tended to slump down. This put strain on the joints of her lower back and pelvis, making her lower back ache. I advised her to sit with her lower back supported by a pillow, or with her bottom tucked well into the back of an upright, supportive, firm chair and her feet on a foot stool with her knees bent.

I advised Susie to do pelvic tilt exercises (see page 59) and showed her alternative ways of sitting (see page 14) and the correct way to stand (see page 12). The three rules of good posture became her catchcry: tummy in, bottom under, shoulders back. I also encouraged her to take an appropriate exercise class. Two weeks later, she showed great improvement.

one-sided upper back pain
or rib pain

Another common complaint during the later stages of pregnancy (30+ weeks) is upper back pain and rib pain. This pain is usually experienced on one side, just under or along the ribcage. It is either a constant or intermittent pain, coming and going according to the woman's posture, and generally worsens when sitting down, or at the end of the day.

This type of pain is due mainly to pressure exerted on the ribs by the growing baby. The uterus, as it enlarges, pushes upward as well as outward, placing pressure on the nerves, muscles and organs in the upper back area.

easing the pain

Certain stretches and positions can help alleviate this discomfort. They can be performed safely as often as you like, and particularly when the pain is acute. In addition, do a few shoulder circles (see page 50) every hour or so. And if you're at home, assume the yoga stretch position for several minutes on the floor or on your bed (see page 63).

Standing side stretch

1 Stand facing a wall. Position your feet comfortably apart, about 60 centimetres away from the wall.

2 Stretch your arms high above your head and lean against the wall. Keep your back straight, trying not to arch your lower back.

3 Place the arm on the painful side up and across the other arm, with your palms flat against the wall. Hold for about 10–20 seconds to give your side a good stretch.

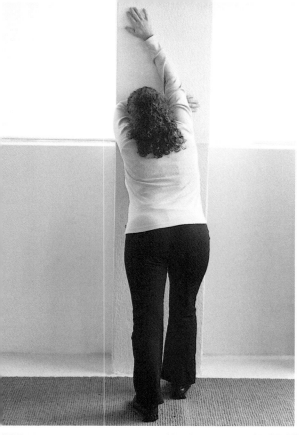

*Left: Standing side stretch –
this eases upper back pain*

*Bottom: The lying side stretch
can also reduce the discomfort
of upper back pain*

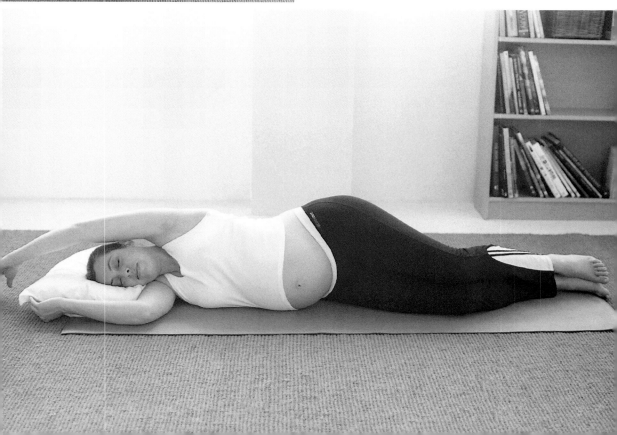

Sitting upper back/rib stretch

1 Sit as straight as possible in a chair at a desk or table. You can even lean forward slightly.

2 Lean your elbows on the desk or table and stretch your body upwards.

Lying side stretch

1 Before sleeping or when resting, lie on your side with the painful side uppermost and your legs in a comfortable position.

2 Stretch the upper arm over your head and hold for 10–20 seconds, then release.

groin pain

Pain in the groin area is usually experienced as a one-sided 'stitch-like' pain when walking too quickly, changing position too quickly, or when coughing or sneezing. It usually passes after a short while. Groin pain is distinct from pubic symphysitis (see page 78); groin pain disappears after a short time, whereas pubic symphysitis pain does not.

Groin pain is a signal to remind you to move more slowly. It is caused by a spasm in the round ligament, which attaches the uterus to the groin area. There is a round ligament on each side of your uterus, anchoring it in place. The pain is completely harmless and is not associated with increased risk of miscarriage or pre-term labour.

easing the pain

Slow down! Move slowly from one position to another. When you feel a cough or a sneeze coming on, try to brace (pull in) your tummy muscles and bend your knees. This can prevent that stitch-like pain from occurring.

case studies

problem: At 35 weeks, Fay complained of a pain in her right side, along her ribs. Sometimes it was sharp, sometimes a dull ache. It was usually sharp towards the end of the day, after she had been sitting at her desk, and she felt the dull ache when she was in bed.

cause: Fay's uterus was probably exerting pressure on the nerves, muscles and organs in her upper rib area.

treatment: A series of a daily stretches (see pages 74–76) would ease her pain. She was very relieved to learn that the pain was likely to disappear altogether when her baby 'dropped' (moved further into the pelvis).

*   *   *

problem: At 32 weeks, almost every time Katharine went shopping and had to use a trolley, she would get a severe 'stitch-like' pain in her groin. It was usually on her right side, but once it was on both sides.

cause: The pushing and pulling action associated with using some of the sticky-wheeled trolleys in her local supermarket was causing the pain.

treatment: Katharine needed to find a trolley that ran smoothly, or reduce the amount of shopping she did at once. If possible, she needed someone to help her shop. Her pain eased with these modifications.

If you do experience this pain and it is convenient to do so, lie down and do the following cycling exercise. If it is not convenient, the best thing you can do is try to relax and wait for the pain to pass.

Cycling exercise

1 Lie on your side, keeping the painful side uppermost, and bend the lower knee.

2 Raise your upper leg away from your body and, as if you are riding a bike, 'cycle' it slowly until the stitch eases. Cycle five to six times, then change direction.

pubic symphysitis

While pubic symphysitis is one of the most common causes of distressing pain in pregnancy, it is often not recognised or treated effectively. The symptoms include either pain and tenderness over the pubic joint – low down in the centre of the groin – pain on one side of the lower back, pain radiating into the right or left groin and inner thigh, or a combination of all of these. It can be felt as a sharp pain or a dull ache, but what differentiates this condition from other lower back pain is that it increases as the pregnancy progresses, and certain movements can make the pain worse. It can become quite debilitating unless diagnosed and treated correctly.

Pubic symphysitis is caused by the laxity of the ligaments and joints of the pelvis, in turn caused by pregnancy-related hormonal changes. In many women, the joint at the front of the pelvis – the pubic symphysis joint (see diagram, page 56) – softens and separates to such an extent that it causes imbalance around the pelvis. Walking and other similar one-sided 'up and down' movements cause friction at this joint, and

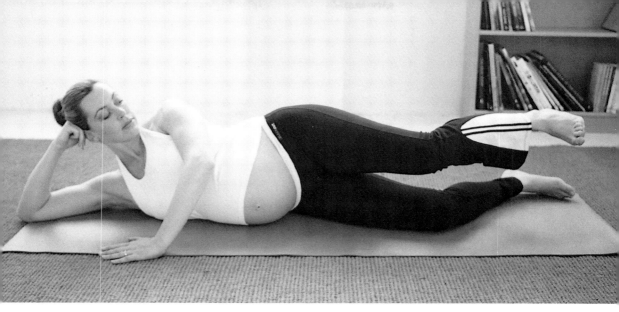

Cycling exercise

it becomes inflamed. The same kind of inflammation can occur in the sacroiliac joints at the back of the pelvis, where it usually leads to one-sided back pain.

Provided your doctor or midwife has given you an assurance that all is well medically, you can relieve this pain by modifying certain movements and/or wearing a special support belt.

easing the pain

When getting into bed, sit on the edge of the bed, press your knees tightly together, then in one movement lie down on your side while lifting your legs up, always remembering to keep your knees together (see page 22).

When rolling from side to side in bed, press your knees together and turn. Do not roll with your knees apart or one at a time.

When getting out of bed, roll onto your side, keeping your knees together and bent. Lower your feet to the floor as you push yourself up to the sitting position. Do not attempt to pull yourself up from lying on your back (see page 22).

Ensure that your weight is evenly distributed over your hips, knees and feet when getting into and out of a chair or car. When you sit down, ensure that you can feel the chair at the back of your legs, then press your knees together and slowly lower yourself into the chair.

When arising from a chair, press your knees together and push yourself up slowly to the standing position, using both hands for assistance.

things to avoid

- Sitting on sofas or soft chairs, as these do not provide adequate support for your pelvic joints or back muscles.
- Using stairs. When this is not possible, take them one at a time, sideways.
- Taking large steps when walking.
- Walking as a form of exercise.

If the pain has not decreased after a week of modifying your movements in this way, you will probably benefit from wearing a special support belt. This can be obtained from the physiotherapy department of most obstetric units at women's hospitals, or from a women's health physiotherapist (see Resources, page 126). Once the physiotherapist has confirmed that the condition is indeed pubic symphysitis, you will be fitted with an appropriate belt, which will decrease the friction in the pubic joint and the lower back joints and give you support around this area.

Spinal adjustments such as chiropractic or osteopathic treatments are not advisable for this condition – it is rest and modifying certain movements that will ease the pain.

It's also important to be aware that certain positions in labour may exacerbate the problem and cause further pain after delivery. These include lying on your back with your legs pulled up and out too far, or side-lying with your top leg pulled right up. Semi-reclining or side-lying with a minimal pull on the hips is acceptable.

If you have pubic symphysitis, inform your doctor and the delivery staff so they can help you with modified delivery positions.

TEN TIPS FOR RELIEVING THE SYMPTOMS OF PUBIC SYMPHYSITIS

1 Avoid twisting your body when reaching for something.

2 Avoid standing with your body weight on one leg only. Stand with equal weight on both feet.

3 Avoid sitting with crossed legs or in the tailor position (the ankle of one leg resting on the knee of the other leg). If you are sitting on a chair, sit symmetrically, with your weight evenly distributed on your hips, knees and feet.

4 When turning from one side to another in bed, keep your knees pressed tightly together. If you sleep with a pillow between your knees, press your knees together to hold the pillow in place when turning, or remove the pillow while turning, then replace.

5 Avoid lifting and carrying heavy objects, especially a heavy shoulder bag.

6 Avoid vacuuming.

7 Adapt your stride length to your pain level: walk with small steps when you feel pain.

8 Take one step at a time when walking up or down stairs. Ideally, walk sideways.

9 When getting into the car, sit down on the seat then bring your legs into the car with your knees and feet together.

10 Sex in the supine (lying on your back) position may cause pain. Try other positions, for example, the side-lying position.

case study

problem: At about 37 weeks, Julie was experiencing pain in her right and left groin and tenderness around her pubic bone. She found the pain most acute when walking, rolling over in bed and trying to get into and out of the car. The pain had been getting gradually worse over the previous four weeks and she felt she could not cope with three more weeks of it. When I palpated her pubic bone, she almost leapt off the bed. She also had a slight limp when walking.

cause: This was a clear case of pubic symphysitis.

treatment: Julie started wearing a support belt to give the joints around her pelvis greater stability and so decrease the movement between them. As soon as she put on the belt for the first time and walked to the end of the room and back, she had a look of amazement and relief on her face. She had no limp and very little pain. She wore the belt at all times, loosening it a little when wearing it to bed. I showed her the correct way to get into and out of bed (see page 22) and the car (see page 25), and how to move correctly from sitting to standing, keeping her weight evenly distributed over her hips and knees at all times, and avoiding any one-sided movement.

leg cramps and swelling

foot and calf muscle cramps

A cramp is the result of a muscle contracting and remaining contracted for a period of time. Cramps in the feet and calf muscles are very common in pregnancy, especially when you have been asleep or resting. They usually occur when you stretch your legs and point your toes, either consciously or during sleep.

With the increased fluid volume in the body during pregnancy and the slowing of the circulation after periods of inactivity such as sleep, merely stretching your legs in this way can bring on a cramp. To avoid getting cramps, as you stretch out your legs, always remember to flex your feet first (pull your toes toward you), hold in this flexed position for a couple of seconds, then point your toes forward. Keep flexing and pointing several times.

EASING THE PAIN

When a cramp occurs, the quickest way to ease it is to pull your toes up toward you, while keeping your knee as straight as possible. Try to hold your leg in this position until the cramp eases, then point your foot gently, then flex, several times. Alternatively, try to stand up and put weight on your foot, or ask your partner or a friend to push up against your foot. Once the cramp has eased, massage the cramping muscle.

Do the flex/point exercise whenever you are resting, as it is a quick and easy way to relieve aching, tired feet and legs. It also promotes good circulation, thus reducing the incidence of cramping.

swollen feet and legs

During pregnancy, your feet and legs are prone to swelling due to hormone action, fluid retention and hot weather. Ensure that your diet does not contain too much salt.

EASING THE PAIN

Try resting with your legs elevated higher than your heart. While your legs are elevated, flex and point your feet several times. Also, circle your feet clockwise and anti-clockwise a few times. This will help reduce the swelling and aching.

When elevating your legs, it is much more effective for reducing swelling and aching to have them higher than your heart. Just stretching them out in front of you is not really elevating them and although this position may be comfortable, it is not as effective.

Massaging with certain aromatherapy oils is a lovely way of relaxing the feet and legs and may also assist in reducing swelling. Warning: Some aromatherapy oils can be harmful during pregnancy. See the Resources, page 127, for who to contact for more information.

You can also ease the discomfort of swelling by:

- making sure you wear comfortable shoes;
- wearing support pantyhose, especially if you have to stand for long periods of time; and
- drinking plenty of water.

Although having swollen feet and legs is common in pregnancy, especially in hot weather or with prolonged standing, the swelling should reduce after a night's rest or sleep. If it persists or also appears in your hands, contact your doctor or midwife, as this can be a sign of high blood pressure.

case study

problem: At 28 weeks, Maria had aching and 'restless' legs, mainly in the evening. She described it as a tired, heavy feeling in her upper legs. Sometimes, while she was in bed, her legs were 'jumpy'.

cause: A possible explanation was that due to increased blood and fluid volume in Maria's body, her legs began to feel heavier than usual, especially after standing for most of the day. When she lay down, her circulation slowed and the 'achy' feeling would begin. Hormonal changes were also a contributing factor.

treatment: First, Maria needed to make sure her shoes were comfortable and supportive. Completely flat shoes do not give the foot adequate support, and high heels can be the cause of an aching back and legs. I advised Maria to wear comfortable, supportive shoes, or consider using arch supports.

Secondly, since Maria's job meant she was standing most of the day, I advised her to wear support pantyhose. These support the blood vessels in the legs and help prevent that aching, swollen feeling.

Finally, it was important for Maria to do regular exercises during the day to get the blood moving. When getting into bed, she should spend a few minutes flexing, pointing and circling her feet to help decrease the aching and also the restless leg sensation.

carpal tunnel syndrome

This syndrome is not as dreadful as it might sound, but it certainly prevents some women from doing normal, everyday activities.

The increase in blood volume and fluid retention in the body during pregnancy can cause nerve compression in the wrist area. This sometimes causes pain in one or both wrists; swelling, tingling or numbness in the fingers; or a combination of these symptoms. It tends to be worse at night or when sleeping, and can either affect women quite severely or very mildly.

easing the pain

Applying ice or an ice pack to your wrists every morning and evening for approximately 20 minutes at a time can bring temporary relief. Another remedy is elevating your hands at night-time.

If symptoms persist, or worsen, it is best to seek physiotherapy advice and treatment in the form of specially made splints or a compression bandage. These hold the wrist in a neutral position and offer relief. Carpal tunnel syndrome usually fades away some time after the baby is born, although the wrist supports may still need to be worn for several weeks post-natally. If the symptoms still persist, see your doctor or physiotherapist.

frequency

Frequency is the medical term for needing to pass urine more than usual. In the early stages of pregnancy, it is hormonal changes that lead to frequency. Then, as you progress in your pregnancy and your baby

case study

problem: Maddy was 36 weeks pregnant when she began experiencing pain and swelling in her right arm and a little less pain in her left arm.

The pain had started as a tingling sensation in her fingers, progressed to numbness in the fingers and then swelling in the hand and arm. It had become so bad that she could no longer safely grasp a cup in her right hand. The symptoms worsened as the day progressed and were at their worst at night.

cause: After checking her hands and neck to rule out other possible causes, it was clear that Maddy had carpal tunnel syndrome.

treatment: Maddy was fitted with special splints that would take the pressure off her wrist by keeping it in a neutral position. She wore the right-hand splint for most of the day and night and the left-hand splint for a few hours during the day. After a week her left hand had improved, but she still felt some pain and swelling in her right hand.

Maddy kept wearing the splint for several weeks to prevent the pain from worsening after childbirth – occasionally the symptoms can return or deteriorate if the affected wrist is being used for weight-bearing activities, such as holding a baby.

keeps growing within the uterus, there is increased pressure on your bladder. This means that you need to empty your bladder far more often than you may have done before pregnancy. However, you will probably pass less urine, or you may also leak a little urine when you sneeze or cough.

easing the discomfort

There is no remedy for frequency – it is just a normal part of pregnancy that virtually every woman experiences. The best advice is to go to the toilet whenever you need to. Keep drinking plenty of fluids, preferably water, and do pelvic floor exercises as often as you can every day (see page 57). Your desire to run to the toilet so often should settle down after you have given birth.

If you experience pain when you pass urine, however, see your doctor – you may have a bladder infection.

varicose veins and haemorrhoids

Painful, aching legs and bluish, prominent veins in the legs, particularly behind the knees, are common signs of varicose veins. But varicose veins can also occur in the vulval and anal areas, leading to what are called vulval varicosities and haemorrhoids. These can be painful and you should try to avoid them if possible.

The occurrence of these varicosities usually runs in the family, so if your mother or father has varicose veins, the likelihood that you will have them is increased. Varicosities occur as a result of hormonal changes and due to the pressure of the growing uterus on the blood vessels in the pelvic area.

easing the effects

Here are some general suggestions to help prevent or ease varicose veins:

- Avoid prolonged standing if you possibly can.
- Do foot/leg circulatory exercises whenever you are sitting or lying down.
- It helps to wear support stockings or pantyhose, but these can be a bit hot in summer. If varicose veins do run in your family, try to persist in wearing support stockings for as long as possible during your pregnancy.
- Put your feet up or elevate your legs whenever you get the opportunity.

Varicose veins that appear during pregnancy usually disappear once the baby is born. In some cases, they remain and increase with subsequent pregnancies.

If you develop vulval varicosities, make sure you do as many pelvic floor exercises as you can manage each day. If this condition is causing you pain, try wearing a sanitary pad pressed against the area with snug-fitting briefs (not bikini-style underpants) to give some relief.

If you are suffering from haemorrhoids during your pregnancy, it may be due to straining on the toilet due to your changing bowel habits. Make sure you exercise regularly, drink plenty of water, and check that you are eating enough roughage in your diet to avoid constipation. When opening your bowels on the toilet, try to squat rather than sitting back or straight – the squatting position is much more effective than sitting (see over for the correct sitting position). Consult your doctor if the constipation continues or the haemorrhoids become very painful or bleed. Resting off your bottom will also offer relief when sitting (see over).

Correct sitting position on the toilet

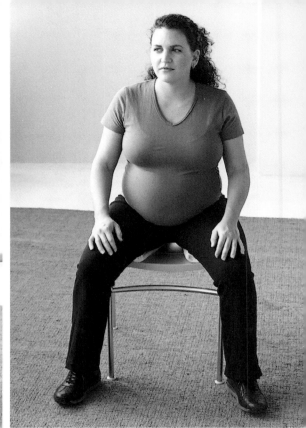

Sitting on rolled towels can provide relief from haemorrhoid pain

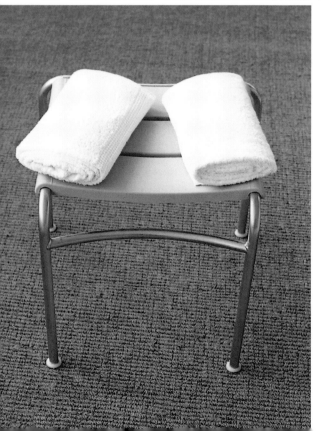

Correct sitting position on the toilet

1 Sit on the toilet with your knees apart.

2 Keeping your back straight, lean your upper body forward and rest your elbows on your knees.

Relief from haemorrhoid pain

1 Place one rolled towel under each buttock and thigh.

2 Sit with the rolled towels under your thighs, so that your bottom is not touching the chair.

forgetfulness, mood swings and sleep disorders

Believe it or not, these conditions are very real and experienced by the majority of women during pregnancy. Hormones are the major cause.

forgetfulness and mood swings

Hormonal changes, along with apprehension – the conscious and sub-conscious mind thinking of the developing baby – can cause you to be a little less alert and perceptive than you might normally be.

Mood swings, sometimes from euphoric happiness to sudden tears, are common. You are not going mad! They will usually settle down after childbirth. So, explain to your partner and your friends that during this time you need consideration and understanding, not criticism.

Accept the hormonal changes taking place in your body. Don't try to fight them. Try to work around forgetfulness by using a notebook or diary to write down everything you need to remember on a day-to-day basis.

Try not to get frustrated. This unusual state will pass, as will most of the other associated symptoms of pregnancy. Whenever I give parent education classes, the looks on couples' faces are of utter relief when they realise they are not the only ones experiencing these symptoms.

insomnia

Not being able to sleep, or waking very early in the morning is a common complaint among pregnant women, particularly those in the third trimester. This can be very frustrating, but try not to let it upset you – after all, once your baby is born, this will be your normal routine for quite a while. Perhaps this is nature's way of preparing you for life with a newborn.

nightmares

Many women experience nightmares towards the end of their pregnancy. They are disturbing and are probably due to subconscious anxieties about the baby and the associated changes to your lifestyle. These, too, will pass. Try relaxation techniques to calm yourself, or just get up and write down the things that may be bothering you. This may help you to release anxieties and make you feel a little calmer before going back to sleep.

heartburn and indigestion

Heartburn and indigestion are also commonly experienced during pregnancy. Hormonal changes cause the softening and loosening of the sphincter muscle in the oesophagus, which, combined with the pressure the growing uterus exerts upwards against the stomach, sometimes means that food and gastric juices rise after eating.

easing the discomfort

Rather than eating large meals three times a day, try to eat smaller amounts of food more often. Make sure you eat slowly, chew your food well, and avoid spicy and fatty foods. Avoid lying down immediately after eating. If heartburn is a problem at bedtime, try to sleep in a semi-upright position, using several pillows to prop yourself up.

Drinking milk as an antacid, sipping peppermint tea and eating ginger are all said to help relieve this problem. Check with your doctor or midwife as to which antacids are safe to take.

Bleeding gums

Hormones are responsible for the softening of the gums during pregnancy, and the increased blood volume in the body makes them a little swollen. You may find that your gums bleed when you brush your teeth. It is important to visit your dentist when you become pregnant, to check whether you have any teeth or gum problems that might deteriorate during pregnancy.

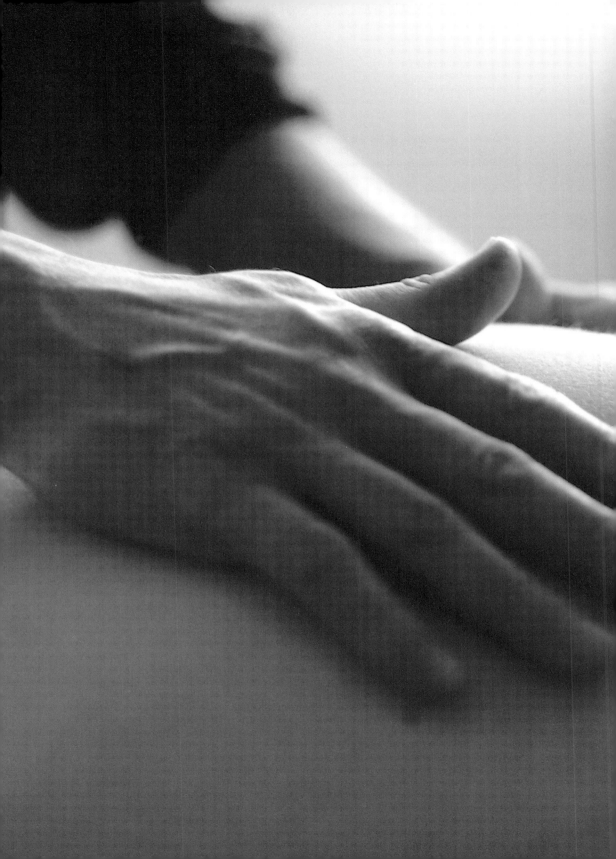

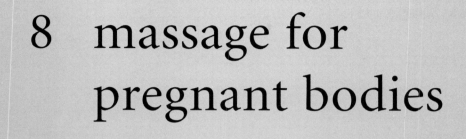

8   massage for pregnant bodies

general massage

Massage is a lovely way of experiencing physical contact in a relaxing, soothing way. It is especially comforting in pregnancy, as your body is so much more stressed and tired. Having your aching, swollen, tired legs and feet massaged is wonderful; and tension in the shoulders and neck can be alleviated with firm, comforting strokes.

All areas of the body can be massaged during pregnancy. Many professional massage therapists are experienced in pregnancy massage. Or, alternatively, your partner can soothe you with some of the following simple, relaxing strokes. If you want to use oil for the massage, try pure sweet almond oil or light olive oil.

When massaging, always work slowly, keeping the hands in contact with the area being massaged at all times. Whether you use firm or soft strokes is up to you – there is no right or wrong way; whatever feels good is good for you.

back massage

Lie on the bed or the floor; you can be in either the side-lying position or the yoga stretch position. Kneeling or sitting comfortably, your partner applies firm, steady strokes up your back on either side of the spine, across your shoulders and down your arms. Your partner should never press on bone – which you will find uncomfortable – but should massage just the soft tissue.

feet and leg massage

Lying on your bed is probably the best position for this massage. Using gentle but firm strokes, your partner massages the tops of your legs with upward strokes, from the knee to the groin.

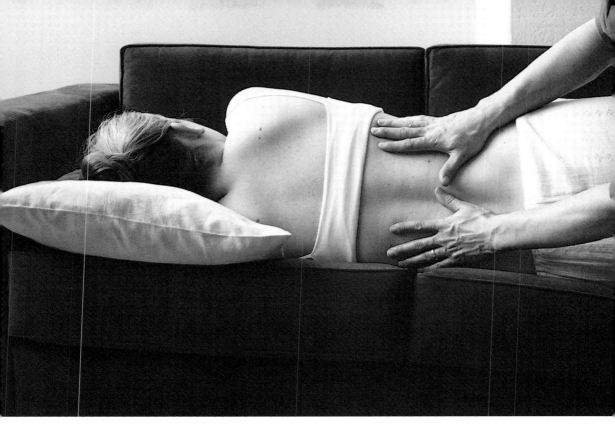

Back massage in the side-lying position

Then, using the same strokes, your partner massages from the ankle to the knee, paying particular attention to the calf muscles and perhaps also applying some kneading strokes here.

Next, your partner massages firmly from the heel to the toes, but be guided by how you feel and relay this to your partner. Having your feet massaged is lovely, provided you are not ticklish.

perineal massage

The advantages of perineal massage during pregnancy are numerous and worth the awkwardness at the beginning. The perineum is the section of body between the vagina and the anus. Massaging the perineal area during pregnancy helps to stretch the skin around the bottom of the vaginal opening and the anus to try to reduce the chance of tearing or having to have an episiotomy (cutting and stitching) during labour.

It is also an effective way to prepare yourself for the sensations of stretching and burning as your baby's head comes through the vaginal opening.

Some women feel comfortable about massaging their perineum, others do not. Remember, it is quite safe to do so, it just takes a bit of getting used to. Starting when you are around 34 weeks pregnant is a good time. Use a mirror so that you can see what you are doing, or ask your partner to perform the massage if they are willing and you feel comfortable about it. Take a warm shower or bath beforehand to warm the perineal area and have some lubricant (water-based) or massage oil handy, such as pure almond or vitamin E oil.

how to massage

1 Making sure that your hands are clean, lean back in a comfortable position, preferably against pillows.
2 Using a water-based lubricant, sweet almond or light olive oil, or even saliva, place your thumbs a couple of centimetres inside your vaginal opening. Press down and out to the sides firmly until you feel a slight burning or stinging feeling.
3 Hold this pressure gently for about 60 seconds, or until the area becomes numb.

4 Keep applying pressure and gently massage the area for 1–2 minutes.

5 Try to exert pressure on the lower part of the vaginal opening (closest to the perineum), as this will help soften and stretch the area that may tear during labour.

Start by massaging for as long as you can tolerate, and increase the duration until you can comfortably massage the perineal area for around 10 minutes.

If you massage your perineum every second day, after a few weeks it will have softened and relaxed and you should no longer feel the burning sensation you felt when you first started.

As you massage your perineum you will feel a burning sensation. This is similar to what you will feel when your baby's head appears and stretches the perineum during birth.

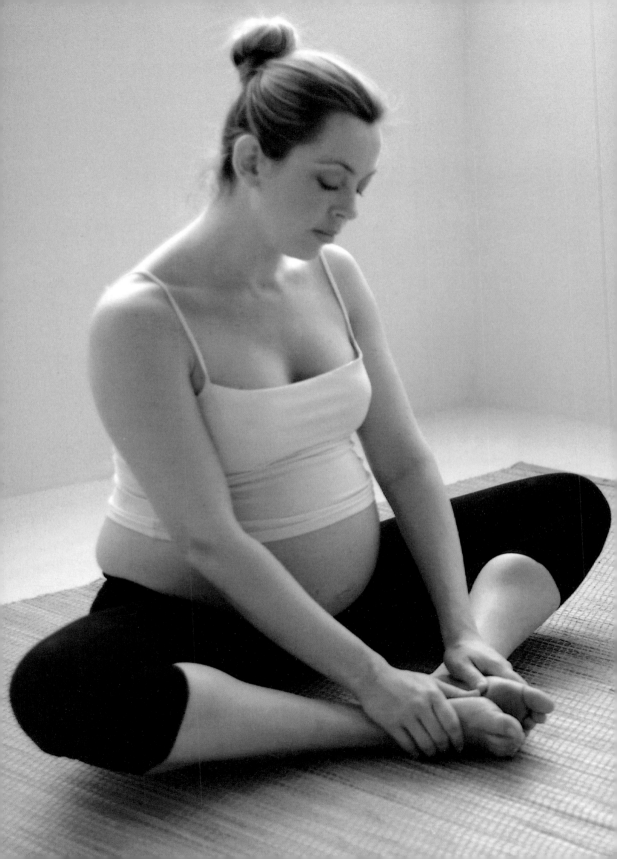

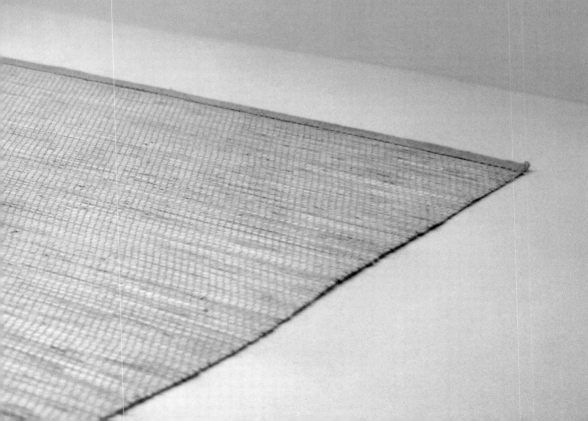

9 relaxation for delivery

relaxation techniques

Practising relaxation techniques at least three times a week, for approximately 20 minutes at a time, will enable you to cope more effectively with stressful situations such as sitting in a traffic jam or visiting the dentist. The more relaxed your mind and body, the easier you will find coping with the most stressful of situations – childbirth.

Let's admit it, childbirth is painful! If you think that labour pains are a slightly stronger form of period pain, think again. Labour is probably the most painful, uncomfortable, difficult experience you will ever have. You will need all the stamina and endurance you can muster.

We usually associate pain with something going wrong – childbirth is probably the only time in life when we associate pain with something going right. It is a positive pain.

Pain in labour comes from the contractions of the uterus, which is a strong and powerful muscle. The uterus contracts to move the baby down the birth canal and to open the cervix. As the contractions become stronger, the pain increases, and this is when relaxation and other coping strategies are used. Any relaxation technique that helps is the right one for you. To know which technique this is, you need to practise each one.

Learning relaxation techniques is relatively simple and once you have mastered the techniques, you will be able to control your body and mind to achieve a sense of peace and control.

Relaxation does not mean sleep, it means being aware of your breathing and how tense your muscles are, and being able to relax them and control your breathing. It means recognising the difference between tense, tight muscles and relaxed, loose muscles; and between everyday inhaling and exhaling, and deep, slow, relaxed breathing. The idea is to be aware of physical tension, and to release it. This takes practice.

muscular relaxation

First, you need to find a position in which you are comfortable and well supported. This can be either a lying or a sitting position. Tense your fingers, hands and arms and hold the tensed position really tight for 5–6 seconds. Now let go. Can you feel the vast difference between tense muscles and relaxed muscles? Repeat this tensing and relaxing, then try it with different parts of your body.

When you are in labour, as the uterus contracts and becomes painful, you will need to be aware of consciously relaxing every other muscle in your body, for example, your jaw, shoulders and hands. By doing this, you will be focusing all your energy onto the uterus and not in 'fighting' the rest of your body.

visualisation

This technique involves using a 'mind picture' or 'thought' as the contraction comes on. One way to use visualisation is to picture what is happening inside your body. Picture the uterus tightening around your baby, pushing it down the birth canal and the cervix opening up. With every contraction, your baby is one step closer to being born. This technique will help you to welcome the contractions, not fight them.

breathing

Breathing is a very powerful relaxation technique. Get into the habit of taking deep, slow breaths, in through your nose and out through your mouth, whenever you are working hard, exercising or in stressful situations. Your muscles will relax and release tension with the exhalation.

In labour, use this deep, slow breathing to cope with the contractions as they become stronger. Your midwife will advise you if and when you need to alter this breathing pattern.

other forms of relaxation

Other things to consider when planning your labour are the use of heat packs – gel-filled packs that can be heated in the microwave – warm towels or warm water. Heat relaxes muscles, so using anything heated to relax you during contractions may give you that little bit of control you need at the time.

The staff in the labour room will be able to supply you with hot towels, but check whether you can bring a heat pack in with you. You can buy these at sports stores and other shops such as Kmart or Target.

Taking a hot shower is another useful coping strategy. Running hot water on your back can be very soothing and empowering.

If you are attending a birth centre, you may be able to use the bath during labour. The staff at the birth centre will advise you whether or not you are suited to delivering in this way.

aromatherapy

Burning your favourite essential oils can help you feel relaxed before, during or after labour. Massage using these aromatic oils can relieve minor aches and pains and swollen feet, and will generally make you feel good. Some essential oils can help prevent stretch marks, and inhaling certain oils during labour can assist with coping strategies.

During your pregnancy, use only the oils considered to be safe, as some essential oils can be harmful for pregnant women (see Resources, page 127). These oils must be not be concentrated. It is advisable to buy a prepared mix suitable for pregnant women, as these will already have been properly diluted.

Aromatherapy can be used during labour, but it is best to seek expert advice about appropriate oils (see Resources, page 127).

RELIEVING SWOLLEN, TIRED FEET

If your feet are aching and swollen, try mandarin, tangerine or cyprus oil, either as a massage oil or by pouring a few drops into a warm foot bath.

Preventing stretch marks

Almond oil combined with a few drops of lavender makes a pleasant massage oil for the hips, tummy, breasts and thighs and will help keep the tightening skin supple and less prone to stretch marks.

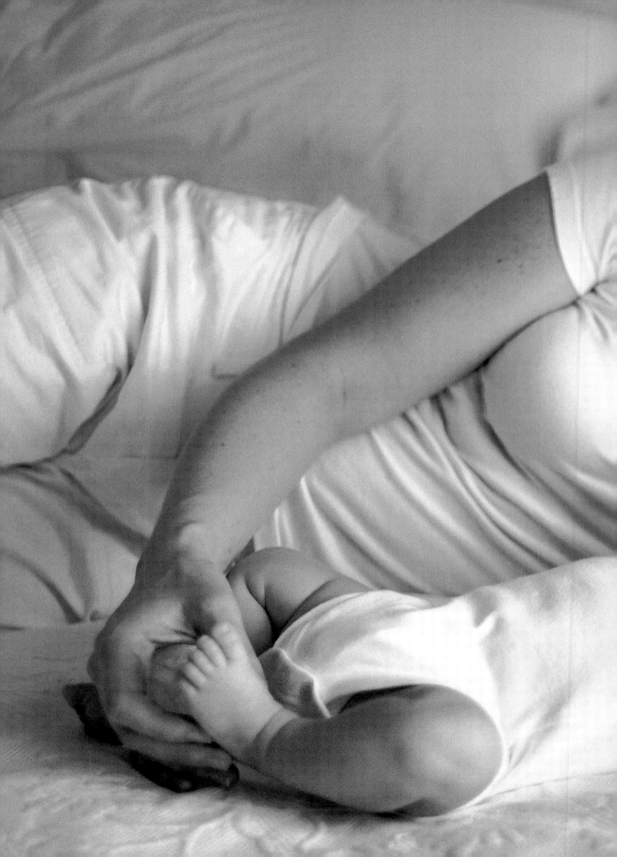

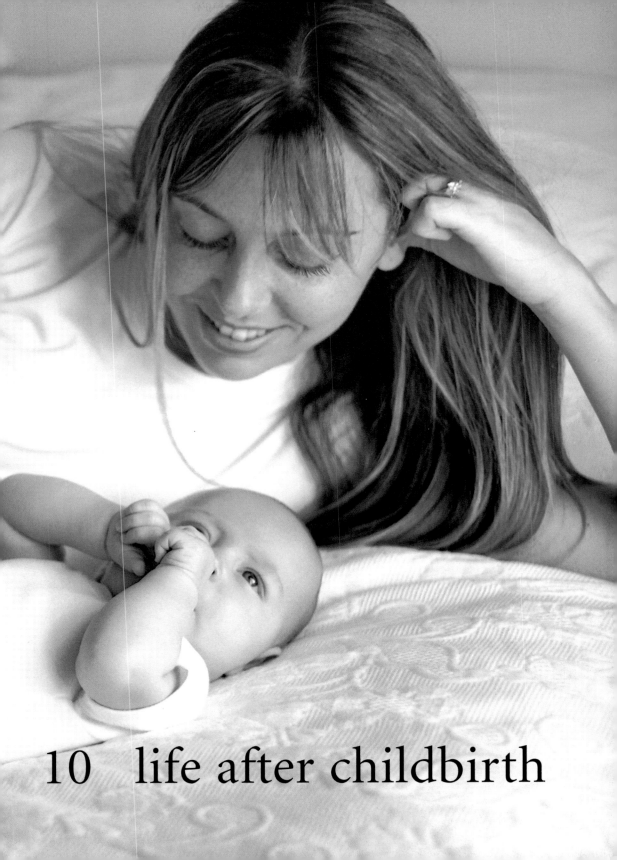

10   life after childbirth

being kind to your recovering body

Once you have had your baby, there are several things to keep in mind as your body recovers. Your ligaments and joints will still be soft for quite a long time after you have given birth. So, in that time, remain conscious of your posture and take care not to strain your back.

It is advisable to begin lying on your tummy 24 hours after giving birth if you have had a vaginal delivery. If you have had a caesarean, you will need to wait a couple of weeks, or until you feel comfortable in that position. Lying on your tummy gives your back a rest and helps with the involution (going down) of the uterus.

Remember, you probably haven't been able to do this for about nine months, so slip a pillow under your tummy, a pillow under your head and shoulders and another pillow under your feet. At first, it may feel strange and uncomfortable, but persevere, as it is completely safe and offers your body the ideal way to relax and fall asleep. Lying in this position for at least 20 minutes per day (or longer if you desire) is beneficial. Be guided by how you feel. If your breasts are sore and swollen (as is most likely the case), place two pillows – one on top of the other – under your head and shoulders and two more, also one on top of the other, under your hips and tummy. This way, there is a nice hollow for your breasts to fit into without putting too much pressure on them.

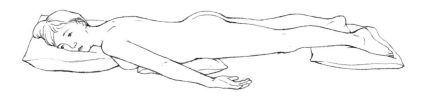

exercise

The best exercise you can do in the immediate post-natal period is walking. Walk for as long as you like and as often as you can, taking your baby in the pram. The fresh air will be enervating and the movement will help your baby go to sleep if he or she is restless. You can start swimming once you have stopped bleeding: while you are still bleeding or experiencing some discharge from your vagina, you may be susceptible to infection from the pool water.

As with any exercise you did during pregnancy, begin with a little at a comfortable level, and build up over time.

If you have had a caesarean delivery, be guided by your medical practitioner as to when you can get into the pool.

You can start specialised fitness classes or low-impact aerobics after the six-week post-natal period. High-impact aerobics classes and high-energy sports such as netball, tennis and squash may affect your milk supply and your ligaments in this post-natal period, so always approach these with caution.

posture and feeding

As a new mother, whether you're breastfeeding or bottle-feeding, you will spend many hours feeding your baby throughout the day and night. The position you adopt is critical if you want to keep upper and lower backache at bay.

Once you arrive home with your baby, set aside a few different areas of the house in which you think you may like to feed your baby, for example, in the loungeroom and bedroom. Important points you should remember are:

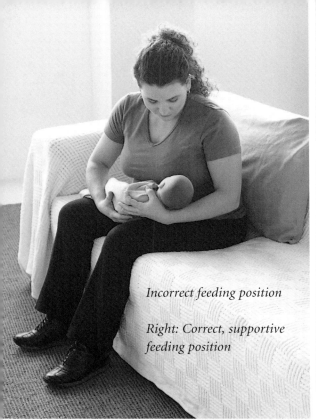

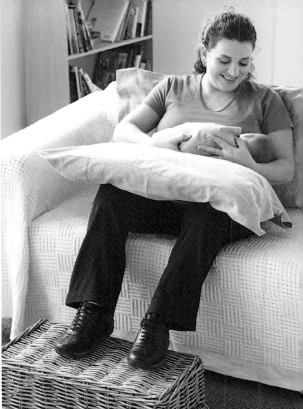

Incorrect feeding position

Right: Correct, supportive feeding position

- sit straight
- support your lower back
- bend your knees comfortably, resting your feet on a stool
- hold your baby chest-to-chest on a pillow on your lap.

If you are sitting in a straight-backed chair, ensure your bottom is tucked well into the chair, and place your feet on a stool, or some other stable object, knees bent and a little higher than your hips. Then you can't stoop over your baby, a major cause of neck and shoulder tightness and pain. A pillow on your lap, under your baby, will bring him or her closer to your breasts and into the chest-to-chest position. If you are sitting on a sofa or soft chair, place a pillow behind your lower back to keep it supported.

To feed your baby while sitting on the floor, sit upright against a wall, your bottom a little away from the wall, your knees bent and feet comfortably apart. Place a pillow on your lap, and position your baby on the pillow.

case study

problem: Emily complained of one-sided upper back and neck pain several days after giving birth to her baby. This is a common post-natal complaint, due to poor feeding posture.

cause: Emily was sitting with her baby at her breast, leaning forward and rotating her head and shoulders to look down at her baby. This meant that every time she fed her baby, she was placing undue strain on her upper back and neck.

treatment: Emily needed to modify her feeding position so that she was sitting with her bottom tucked well into an upright chair, with her back straight, pillow on her lap, and her baby on the pillow. Most importantly, she needed to rest her feet on a foot stool, with her knees bent and elevated slightly higher than her hips. In this position, she was unable to rotate her shoulder or lean forward, her back was relaxed and her pain disappeared. I also advised her to do some mobilising exercises to keep her upper back and shoulder areas flexible (see pages 50–53).

If you prefer feeding on your bed, use the same position, but lean against the bedhead or the wall.

These positions ensure that you cannot lean forward, so your upper back, shoulders and neck will remain relaxed and pain-free. Even so, it's a good idea to do a few shoulder circles and upper back stretches after completing a feed (see page 50). It is far easier to do a few of these simple exercises to prevent problems, rather than dealing with them if or when they arise.

When carrying your baby, alternate the side you carry him or her: one day on your right hip, the next day on your left, and so on. This will help you avoid one-sided lower back and hip pain.

back care

If we all looked after our backs a little more throughout our younger years, very few of us would have back problems later in life. It is very easy to do the right thing by your back if you know how. During pregnancy and in the post-natal period it is especially important.

Wherever possible, ensure that your work areas are at waist-height. This is especially important if you are tall, as most work surfaces and benches are geared to people of average height, requiring you to stoop. If you do chores there, you will soon have backache.

Before buying a change table or bathing table, try out the different ones on the market until you find one that is suitable and reaches to your waist. This will ensure that your back stays straight and that you are not stooping over when tending to your baby. Try to refrain from changing your baby's nappy on the bed, as this is usually much lower than waist-height and will eventually lead to a stiff, sore back.

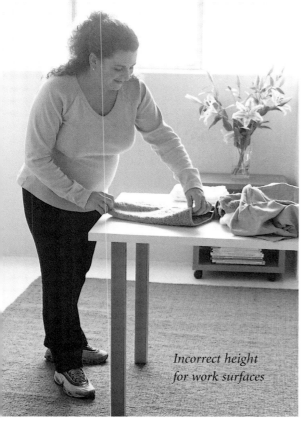

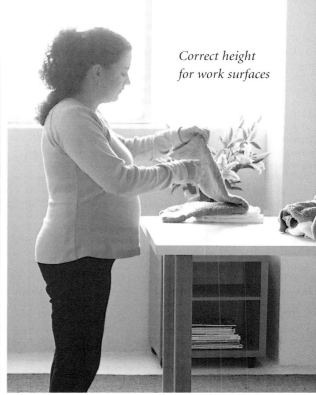

Correct height for work surfaces

Incorrect height for work surfaces

There are countless other household chores that may cause you to stoop and do damage to your back, so think through the different ways you can modify your activities to get the job done while maintaining good posture.

As mentioned in Chapter 7, when you are doing the ironing, ensure that the ironing board is at waist-height. It is also very helpful to use a trolley for your washing basket when hanging out washing so that you avoid carrying a heavy load of wet washing and having to bend down to pick up each article of clothing.

Use an upright vacuum cleaner so that you are not pushing and rotating the body. The barrel-style vacuum cleaner has the potential to cause back strain.

When mopping or sweeping, try to stand upright and do not twist. These are all good life long habits!

baby positions

When putting your baby down to sleep, most child-care professionals recommend that you place baby on his or her back. However, alternating the position of your baby's head each sleep is helpful so that pressure is not exerted more on one side than the other during the first few months. So, for example, if you place your baby in the cot with the back of the head on the mattress, next sleep put him or her down with the head on the right side, then the following sleep, put the head on the left side, and so on. Your baby will most likely find this a comfortable way to adapt to differing sleeping positions.

If you always put your baby down to sleep with his or her head on the same side, or always with the back of the head on the mattress, the head will tend to become a little misshapen. Don't be alarmed if this happens – as the baby keeps growing, the head will even itself out.

Although you should never put your baby down on the tummy to sleep, when he or she is awake, a few supervised minutes on the tummy can be beneficial, as it encourages the baby to lift his or her head and this helps strengthen the neck muscles. Placing the baby over your lap on his or her tummy has the same effect. A few minutes at a time is plenty, or be guided by the baby's reaction. Some babies love the position, others don't and will let you know. Having toys and bumpers – thick, soft sausage-shaped rolls of foam – in the cot is not recommended.

perineal care

If you have had a vaginal delivery, especially with a tear or stitches, your perineum is likely to be sore and swollen. This will have been attended to in hospital, but if you find that your perineal area is still sore and tender after you return home, apply a cold pack for 10–20 minutes at a time, as often as you like. This will help reduce swelling and decrease pain. Another useful hint is to drink plenty of water to dilute your urine – to lessen the stinging sensation of the urine on the perineal area.

When trying to empty your bowels with a sore perineum, try supporting the perineal area with a wad of toilet paper. This provides a counter-pressure and makes it less painful and stressful to have a bowel motion. Keep doing this until the area returns to normal and the pain has gone.

Finally, remember to eat lots of roughage, in the form of bran, cereals, fruit and so on, to avoid becoming constipated, and keep drinking lots of water, especially if you're breastfeeding your baby. Even if you are sore, keep trying to do your pelvic floor exercises; by using these muscles, the sore area will heal more quickly.

While the area is still sore but healing, position a rolled-up towel under each thigh when you sit. This will take the pressure off the perineal area and make sitting a lot more comfortable.

sex after childbirth

Every woman feels different about resuming sexual relations after having a baby. There is no right or wrong time. It is entirely up to you as a couple.

Some women may feel pain in the vaginal area a few weeks after giving birth, but this does subside gradually. If you still feel pain or discomfort after six weeks, have this checked by your doctor, who will make sure everything is healing well. Also, ask your doctor to check the tone of your pelvic floor muscles at your six-week post-natal check.

Remember that you can fall pregnant while breastfeeding, so it may be a good idea to use contraception once you recommence sexual relations. If you are undecided about which contraceptive method to use, again, your doctor or midwife will advise you.

post-natal pelvic floor advice

If you have been doing your pelvic floor exercises throughout your pregnancy, well done, now keep going! If you have not, begin them as soon as possible. Regardless of what type of delivery you have had, you must begin exercising these muscles as soon as possible after the birth and you should continue to do so for the rest of your life.

Why? As discussed in Chapter 6, the hormonal changes during your pregnancy cause softening of your muscles and ligaments. Your pelvic floor muscles soften, the growing baby and uterus exert pressure on the muscles, then, during a vaginal delivery, with the baby coming through them you may have been left with stretched, weak pelvic floor muscles. These muscles will regain tone with time, but they will not be as strong as they were before pregnancy, unless you exercise them. If you do not exercise them they will become weaker and looser every time you have a baby, and this effect is cumulative. You may be lucky and have no symptoms of incontinence in your younger years, but as you grow older and get nearer to the menopause, the likelihood of having problems increases. You may find one day that you are unable to 'hold on', you are not getting to the loo in time, or you are losing a bit of urine when coughing, sneezing or running. This only gets worse, not better!

Another problem discussed in Chapter 6 is prolapse, the 'dropping down' of the uterus, bladder or bowel, which is often the result of very weak pelvic floor muscles and repeated vaginal deliveries. This condition is more commonly seen the closer a woman is to menopause. The damage occurs at childbirth and, with the hormonal changes at menopause, the woman may begin to experience a feeling that something is 'dropping down' or a 'dragging' sensation. Once a woman has reached this point, physiotherapy treatment can reduce symptoms of minor prolapse. However, if left untreated and the condition progresses to severe prolapse, surgery is usually required. Try to avoid this condition – EXERCISE! EXERCISE! EXERCISE THOSE PELVIC FLOOR MUSCLES!

If you have any sign of incontinence and pelvic floor exercises do not seem to help, contact a continence advisor or physiotherapist specialising in incontinence, for further advice and treatment. If you have symptoms of prolapse, it is best to see a gynaecologist.

good bladder habits

The bladder can hold between 300 and 600 millilitres of urine and needs emptying four to six times daily, and sometimes once during the night. During pregnancy, the pressure of the uterus on the bladder causes you to want to empty it much more frequently and, as a result, you pass less urine than usual. This is normal, but should not persist after you have given birth.

The post-natal period is the time to focus on good bladder habits. Follow the advice below and you will decrease the likelihood of having bladder control problems later in life.

- Drink at least eight glasses of water a day (more if breastfeeding).
- Reduce your caffeine intake, for example, cola drinks, coffee and tea.
- Go to the toilet only when you really need to, and not 'just in case'.

If you find you are going to the toilet more than six times a day, try to re-train your bladder by ignoring the first signal telling you to go. Focus your mind on something else. Don't think about the toilet. When you get the next urge to go, do so. By ignoring that first urge, you can gradually re-train your bladder to give you the signal to go only when it is full, not partially full. The one exception is going to the toilet before going to bed at night. You should go then, but only if you really need to.

emotions

Once your baby has been born, the levels of the hormone relaxin in your body begin to decrease and other hormonal changes occur. It is important in the six or so weeks following delivery not to expect things to return to the way they were before you were pregnant, both emotionally and physically. Never expect to be a 'supermum' – it is unrealistic. A baby takes up a lot of your physical and emotional energy and, although having a newborn baby is a joyous event, it is a very difficult time.

Do not even try to manage housework, cooking and looking after the baby. It is not possible to be perfect; just do what you can, when you can, and make sure you look after your own wellbeing. If anyone offers help with cooking, shopping or housework, say yes. Delegate chores if people are willing to do them. You cannot do everything and remain sane.

Try to set aside at least one hour per day for yourself alone. Exercise, read, have a bath, do your nails, relax – anything, as long as it is uninterrupted and solely for yourself. It is also important that your partner has realistic expectations of you in those first few weeks. If you do not have a partner, ask a friend or member of your family to help.

'the blues' and post-natal depression

At around three days after delivery, many women begin to experience feelings of sadness and are easily brought to tears. This is usually due to the hormonal changes taking place at the time. The mood swings may last for a couple of days or weeks. They will then fade away.

Initially, there is great excitement when the baby is born; you may have lots of people congratulating you and you may feel wonderful. Then you go home with the new baby and the hard work begins. You will have broken sleep patterns and you will be tired as you try to manage your new life. It is not an easy time.

However, it does become easier once you establish routines. After a few weeks, things begin to become familiar, patterns and routines become more established and you will generally feel more in control.

If, however, after a few weeks, you still feel depressed and have thoughts of harming yourself or your baby, seek help. You may have post-natal depression. Speak to your doctor or early childhood nurse. They can help and you will get better. It can be as easy as talking to the right person and having your fears and concerns dealt with appropriately.

Never feel embarrassed or shy about voicing your concerns or seeking help. The early childhood centre in your area will also offer helpful advice.

life after a caesarean delivery

In my experience of talking to and treating pre- and post-natal women, far too many women who have had a caesarean delivery are disappointed and distressed at not having had a vaginal delivery. Try not to be! The most important thing about childbirth is to deliver your baby safely, not the method by which you bring your baby into the world.

case study

problem: When Nicole's first baby was eight weeks old, she came to see me to have her tummy muscles checked. After talking with her for a few minutes, she became teary and said that she felt 'overwhelmed' and thought that she hated her baby at times. She felt she was not in control, she was not getting much sleep and did not feel like doing anything or going out. She felt hopeless and sad, couldn't eat and was anxious. And, to make matters worse, she didn't have much support as her family lived overseas.

cause: Nicole was clearly suffering from post-natal depression.

treatment: With her permission, I phoned her doctor, who arranged to refer her to an appropriate counselling service.

You can contact organisations such as Tresillian and Karitane by phone if you have problems with baby settling, feeding, and so on (see Resources, page 125). Physiotherapy departments and midwives at the hospital at which you gave birth will always be helpful, as will the lactation staff. Don't ever be shy about asking for help.

If circumstances are such that a caesarean is needed, so be it. These operations are not performed for fun; they are necessary in most cases.

A caesarean delivery is simply a different experience to a vaginal delivery. Post-natally, you will probably need more assistance with moving, getting in and out of bed and so on, compared with someone who has had a vaginal delivery.

Regardless of the type of delivery, most women experience pain and discomfort for two or three days, just in different areas. If you have had a vaginal delivery, you will experience pain in the vaginal and perineal areas. If you have had a caesarean delivery, it will be abdominal pain.

Usually, it takes around six weeks after delivery to be able to function 'normally'. It takes that long to heal internally, not just externally. So don't do anything too strenuous until after that time, and even then, take care.

feeding difficulties

Many women experience sore, hard breasts when the breastmilk first comes in at about the third or fourth day after childbirth, but this should not persist once the baby begins feeding properly. Although breastfeeding is a normal, natural process, it is not always easy and can be quite painful initially. The midwives can help you establish the correct feeding technique before you leave hospital. If you find you have any ongoing feeding problems, contact a breastfeeding hotline for advice (see Resources, page 126).

Whether you decide to breastfeed or bottle-feed, the choice is yours. You will be encouraged by doctors, nurses and midwives to breastfeed unless there is a reason that you cannot, but whatever the reason, if you decide you want or need to bottle-feed, you should do so without feeling guilty. You are the mother, it is up to you to decide.

case study

problem: Two days after Lynne delivered her baby by caesarean section she was worried that she would 'burst' the stitches when trying to get out of bed. She was also distressed at the amount of pain she was experiencing.

cause: Any incision, small or large, over the abdominal area will result in pain. This is because we use our abdominal muscles to do almost any movement, for example, reaching for the phone, rolling over in bed, getting up from lying to sitting, sitting to standing, coughing, laughing, sneezing, and so on. Although it hurt doing these activities, Lynne wouldn't be doing any damage to the abdominal area or incision site. The problem was solely a pain-management one.

treatment: When coughing or sneezing, Lynne would need to support her abdominal area by holding a pillow firmly against her tummy, while bending her knees. When getting out of bed, rolling slowly onto her side first, before pushing herself up, would be easier than pulling up into the sitting position from lying. Finally, she was not do any strenuous activities such as vacuuming, heavy lifting or carrying for approximately six weeks.

Lynne's pain and discomfort gradually decreased over the next few weeks.

Persistently sore nipples are due mainly to incorrect attachment of the baby's mouth on the areola area. Make sure that your baby is feeding correctly before leaving hospital. If the soreness continues, or your breasts become lumpy or hot, see your midwife or early childhood nurse; they will advise if it is necessary to see your doctor.

If you are diagnosed with mastitis, you will probably need a course of antibiotics. Along with antibiotics, physiotherapy treatment, in the form of ultrasound to the breast, can help alleviate the symptoms.

sore coccyx

Some women experience a sore coccyx (tailbone) after delivery, which is often due to the position they adopted during labour. It usually disappears several weeks after the delivery.

If pain in your coccyx persists for several months, or you have had a previous injury to this area, it may help to have it checked by a doctor via X-ray, and you may then benefit from some physiotherapy exercises.

Correct posture when sitting is important (see page 14). Sitting on rolled-up towels will give you some relief during the painful stage.

abdominal muscle separation

Your post-childbirth abdominal separation will most likely have been checked by the physiotherapist at the hospital or by the early discharge sister at your home. Usually, if the separation is greater than three finger-widths, it is advisable to wear an abdominal binder, which will help keep the abdominal and back muscles supported, for a time. The binder should be fitted by the hospital physiotherapist and you should also begin the appropriate abdominal strength exercises (see page 39).

Once the separation decreases, you can dispense with the binder, but keep doing the exercises, increasing them as instructed.

checking your abdominal separation

Lie on your bed or on the floor with your knees bent. Lift your head and shoulders and, using your fingers, feel the area just above and below your belly button. Run your fingers across and you will feel a hollow space between the muscles. This is the abdominal separation. See how many finger-widths fit across this dip.

Exercise daily for one week, then measure the separation again to see if it has narrowed. Continue exercising until the gap is one finger-width. If you are wearing a binder you can stop once the separation is two finger-widths. Your physiotherapist can monitor your progress.

epidural back pain

A lot of women have commented to me that they experienced back pain several days after having had an epidural and that they think the epidural was responsible. This is highly unlikely (unless there is visible bruising).

This type of pain is usually due to the position you were in while you were under the effect of the epidural, when you were unable to feel if you were in an uncomfortable position.

Being in an unusual position for a couple of hours will inevitably lead to aches and pains once sensation returns. If you had normal sensation, you would have moved yourself around but, as you were unable to, the result is muscle or joint pain for the next few days.

resources

The following services are all available to the new mother with questions, issues or problems regarding herself or her baby. They are very helpful, informative and non-judgemental.

SIDS

If you have any questions at all about SIDS you can visit SIDS and kids online at www.sidsaustralia.org.au or phone:

ACT	(02) 6287 4255
NSW	(02) 9681 4500 or 1800 651 186
Hunter region	(02) 4969 3171
VIC	(03) 9822 9611 or 1800 240 400
TAS	(03) 6431 9488 or 1800 625 675
QLD	(07) 3849 7122 or 1800 628 648
SA	(08) 8363 1963 or 1800 656 566
WA	(08) 9474 3544 or 1800 199 466
NT	(08) 8948 5311

KARITANE

NSW	24-hour Careline (02) 9794 1852 or 1800 677 961
VIC	Karitane Children's Centre (03) 9457 2930
QLD	Riverton Centre (07) 3860 7111
WA	Ngala Family Resource Centre (08) 9368 9368 or 1800 111 546

TRESILLIAN FAMILY CARE CENTRES

NSW	(02) 9787 5255 (Rural NSW & ACT 1800 637 357)
ACT	Queen Elizabeth II Family Centre (02) 6205 2333
VIC	Queen Elizabeth Centre (03) 9549 2777
	O'Connell Family Centre (03) 9882 2326
	Tweddle Child & Family Health Service (03) 9689 1577
TAS	Parenting Centre (03) 6233 2700 or 1800 808 178 (AH)
QLD	Riverton Centre (07) 3860 7111
SA	Torrens House (08) 8303 1530
WA	Ngala Family Resource Centre (08) 9368 9368 or 1800 111 546

BREASTFEEDING

For help with breastfeeding visit the Australian Breastfeeding Association (ABA, formerly the Nursing Mothers' Association) website at www.breastfeeding.asn.au or call one of the breastfeeding helplines:

ACT/southern NSW	(02) 6258 8928
NSW	(02) 9639 8686
VIC	(03) 9885 0653
southern TAS	(03) 6223 2609
northern TAS	(03) 6331 2799
QLD	(07) 3844 8977
SA & NT	(08) 8411 0050
WA	(08) 9340 1200

PARENT HELP LINES

These are confidential telephone counselling and referral services for parents. Calls are answered by trained counsellors who have experience in helping families deal with problems. Call:

ACT	Parent Support Service (02) 6278 3996
NSW	Parentline (Centacare) 13 20 55
VIC	Parent Line 13 22 89
QLD	Parentline 1300 301 300
SA	Parent Helpline 1300 364 100
WA	Parent Line (08) 9272 1466 or 1800 654 432 (outside Perth)

EARLY CHILDHOOD CENTRES

Contact numbers are available in your local telephone book or from your local council.

PHYSIOTHERAPISTS

Call your nearest branch of the Australian Physiotherapy Association to find out how to contact a women's health physiotherapist:

NSW	(02) 8748 1555
VIC	(03) 9429 1799
QLD	(07) 3391 7100
WA	(08) 9389 9211

AROMATHERAPY

For more information on aromatherapy oils and advice for suitable treatments during pregnancy, you can contact the International Federation of Aromatherapists (Australian Branch) Inc. (IFA) at PO Box 786, Templestowe VIC 3106, or info@ifa.org.au or by calling:

Australia-wide	1902 240 125
NSW	Frances Sodaro 0401 201 316
	Rosa Ghidella (02) 9797 0422
northern NSW	Ann George (02) 6584 0027
VIC	Ann Youatt (03) 5962 1912
TAS	Irma Gol (03) 6243 7713
northern QLD	John Monz (07) 4773 2728
WA	Jennifer Jones (08) 9385 3117

A useful book to consult is Allison England's *Aromatherapy and massage for mother and baby: How essential oils can help you in pregnancy and early mother-hood* published in the United Kingdom by Vermilion in 1999 and in the United States by Healing Arts Press in 2000.

To obtain aromatherapy products for suitable for use during pregnancy and labour, contact Professional Aromatherapy Products on (02) 9327 6978.

FURTHER READING

Collins, Mary (ed.) *Women's health through life stages: The physiotherapist's contribution*, Australian Physiotherapy Association (NSW Branch), Sydney, 1987.

England, Allison *Aromatherapy and massage for mother and baby: How essential oils can help you in pregnancy and early motherhood*, Vermilion, London, 1999.

Llewellyn-Jones, Derek *Everywoman: A gynaecological guide for life*, 5th edition, Penguin, Melbourne, 1992.

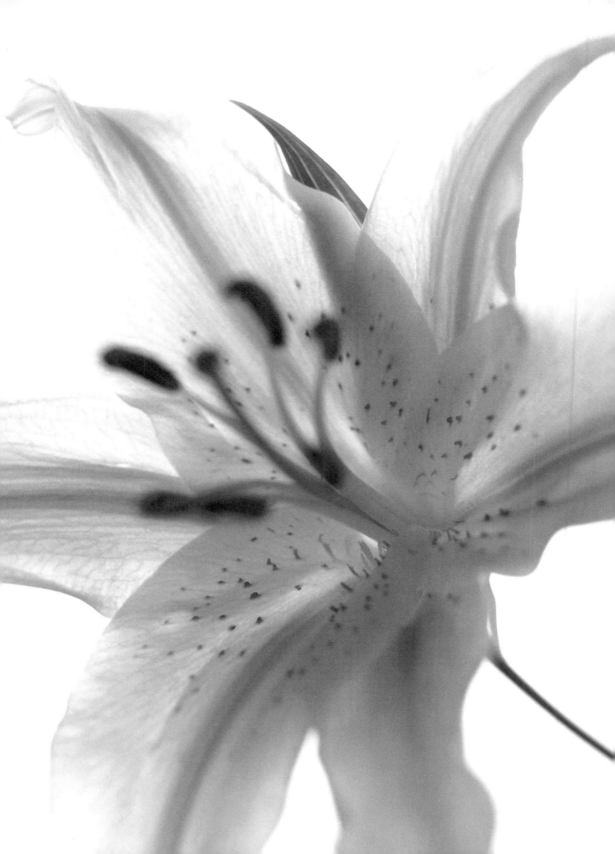

index

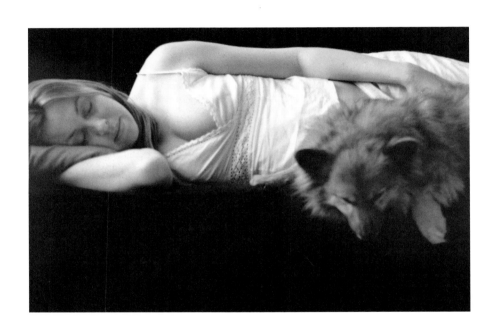